Acromegaly

PATHOLOGY, DIAGNOSIS AND TREATMENT

Acromegaly

PATHOLOGY, DIAGNOSIS AND TREATMENT

Aart Jan van der Lely
Erasmus University Medical Center
Rotterdam, The Netherlands

Albert Beckers
Centre Hospitalier Universitaire de Liège
University of Liège
Liège, Belgium

Adrian F. Daly
Centre Hospitalier Universitaire de Liège
University of Liège
Liège, Belgium

Steven W. J. Lamberts
Erasmus University Medical Center
Rotterdam, The Netherlands

David R. Clemmons
University of North Carolina
Chapel Hill, North Carolina, U.S.A.

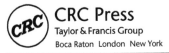

CRC Press
Taylor & Francis Group
Boca Raton   London   New York

CRC Press is an imprint of the
Taylor & Francis Group, an **informa** business

Cover illustrations courtesy of A. Beckers, P. Petrossians, and J. Trouillas. Front cover concept by Stealth Moose Designs.

CRC Press
Taylor & Francis Group
6000 Broken Sound Parkway NW, Suite 300
Boca Raton, FL 33487-2742

First issued in paperback 2019

© 2005 by Taylor & Francis Group, LLC
CRC Press is an imprint of Taylor & Francis Group, an Informa business

No claim to original U.S. Government works

ISBN-13: 978-0-8493-3848-9 (hbk)
ISBN-13: 978-0-367-39258-1 (pbk)

Library of Congress Cataloging-in-Publication Data

Catalog record is available from the Library of Congress

**Visit the Taylor & Francis Web site at
http://www.taylorandfrancis.com**

**and the CRC Press Web site at
http://www.crcpress.com**

Preface

Recent years have seen important advances in nearly all aspects of the management of acromegaly. Molecular and genetic studies have brought us closer to understanding the events that lead to tumorigenesis in sporadic and inherited forms of acromegaly. The criteria for determining disease activity in acromegaly have narrowed in a relatively short period of time and provide a clear yardstick against which we can measure therapeutic efficacy. Long-term outcome studies have shown the undoubted benefits of growth hormone (GH) and insulin-like growth factor-I (IGF-I) normalization in terms of reducing mortality in acromegaly to that of the general population, thus providing an added impetus for seeking strict disease control. Incremental refinements in neurosurgical techniques continue to improve outcomes, particularly when performed by a dedicated pituitary surgeon. Innovations in radiotherapy, such as radiosurgery, also promise to control acromegaly, potentially with a lower attendant risk of adverse events. In addition to the established medical therapies, i.e., long-acting somatostatin analogs and dopamine agonists, a new GH receptor antagonist, pegvisomant, has been introduced, which promises to provide control of IGF-I in nearly all patients. These treatment options, when used either singly or as a part of multimodal therapy, could ensure effective control in all but the most resistant cases of acromegaly.

Acromegaly: Pathology, Diagnosis and Treatment has been written to provide a timely and concise overview of the current management of the disease, and is divided into three broad sections, echoing the title. The first section, *Pathology*, begins with a timeline that details some of the most important events in the history of the management of acromegaly. This is followed by a description of the normal function of the pituitary and GH–IGF-I axis. The first section ends with an overview of the epidemiology, pathophysiology, and pathological complications of acromegaly. The second section, *Diagnosis*, concentrates on the clinical, radiological, and hormonal criteria for diagnosing acromegaly, with particular emphasis being placed on the use of modern GH/IGF-I cut-off levels. *Treatment*, the third section, devotes separate chapters to the relative benefits of the five treatment modalities now available: surgery, somatostatin analogs, a GH-receptor antagonist, dopamine agonists, and radiotherapy.

Acromegaly: Pathology, Diagnosis and Treatment is intended for both specialists and interested general physicians alike, as a broad awareness of the disease is important if it is to be diagnosed and treated as early as possible. This book may also be helpful to endocrinology fellows in training and students at the early stages of their careers, providing information on the care of acromegaly.

Finally, we would like to acknowledge the following for their generosity to us in terms of their time and also for allowing us to reproduce images contained in the book: Dr. Patrick Petrossians of CHU de Liège and Graphmed (Belgium); Dr. Achille Stevenaert of CHU de Liège (Belgium); Mr. Paul Glacken and the Department of Anatomy, Trinity College (Dublin, Ireland); Mr. Vladimir Chichkov (Tampa, Florida, U.S.A.); Dr. K. Kovacs (Toronto, Canada); Dr. J. Trouillas (Lyon, France); Dr. W. de Herder (Rotterdam, The Netherlands); the Ägyptisches Museum, Staatliche Museen zu Berlin (Germany); and Cameraphoto Arte (Venice, Italy). Special thanks to Dr. Serena Durán for her insightful comments on the content and layout of the manuscript. Our gratitude also goes to the team at Dekker/Taylor & Francis for all of their hard work in making this book a reality. In particular, we would like to thank our commissioning editor, Sandra Beberman, for her tenacity and forbearance throughout the process of completing this publication.

Aart Jan van der Lely
Albert Beckers
Adrian F. Daly
Steven W. J. Lamberts
David R. Clemmons

Contents

Section I

PATHOLOGY

1

Acromegaly:
A Historical Timeline

INTRODUCTION

Diseases that significantly alter physical appearance have always aroused human curiosity, and perhaps none more so than those related to stature and growth. To trace the history of acromegaly is to visit many of the most important figures and events within endocrinology, which itself is celebrating the 100th anniversary of the introduction of the word "hormone" by Starling (1). Both the medical and lay communities have always demonstrated fascination with gigantism and acromegaly, although in earlier times this interest was not entirely benign in nature. Fundamental discoveries concerning the pituitary gland and the etiology of acromegaly and gigantism were made in the late 19th and early 20th centuries, paralleling the birth of modern medicine. Indeed, acromegaly played an important role in revealing how the hypothalamus and pituitary dictate peripheral organ function via circulating hormones. The initial treatment of acromegaly with surgery and radiation occurred just as the principles and techniques of neurosurgery and radiotherapy were being laid down for the first time. Each major technological breakthrough, such as the radioimmunoassay, magnetic resonance imaging, and new molecular genetic techniques, has contributed enormously to the way we assess and treat acromegaly today. This historical timeline traces briefly some of the more important persons and milestones related to acromegaly.

PREHISTORY TO IMPERIAL ROME

Accounts of giants and dwarfs can be found in the art and literature of most cultures. The earliest evidence that is suggestive of gigantism and acromegaly comes from thousands of years ago, although the veracity of these accounts is debatable. Most notable among these is the familiar biblical story of the giant Goliath, who reportedly measured "6 cubits and a span," the equivalent of 2.74 meters, over 9 feet. It has been speculated that the ease with which David's slingshot felled Goliath may have been due to a visual defect related to chiasmal impingement by a pituitary adenoma. Unsurprisingly, the biblical description of this encounter is devoid of data to support such a theory; however, as noted by Sheaves (2), a later depiction of the face of Goliath dating from the 18th century arguably bears acromegalic features.

Other ephemeral evidence of acromegaly in distant history has come from ancient Egyptian art, which has also provided accurate depictions of other growth disorders, such as achondroplasia. The pharaoh of the 18th Egyptian dynasty, Amenhotep IV, or Akhenaten, reigned together with his wife Nefertiti during a period that saw major political, religious, and artistic changes, which have led to intense study of this period. Images of Akhenaten and his family differ remarkably from previous pharaonic representations. Akhenaten is typically depicted as having a pendulous abdomen, gynecomastia, and, in some cases, an elongated chin, enlarged lips, and a heavy brow (Fig. 1). While it is possible to ascribe this constellation of signs to acromegaly with associated hypogonadism, this is probably a fanciful modern interpretation. Furthermore, the clinical significance of Akhenaten's "hypogonadal" appearance is questionable, as he fathered six daughters with Nefertiti. It has been suggested that Akhenaten was also the father of Tutenkhaten, later known more familiarly as the pharaoh Tutenkhamun.

From Roman times, the most significant reputed giant was the Emperor Gaius Julius Verus Maximinus, a Thracian who is commonly referred to as Maximinus "Thrax." After overthrowing the existing Emperor Severus Alexander in a military revolt in 235 A.D., Maximinus Thrax ruled until 238 A.D., when he himself was the victim of a similar coup. Maximinus Thrax was of outstanding physical stature (reportedly about 2.6 meters in height) and was said to be capable of astounding feats of strength. The images we have of Maximinus Thrax come predominantly from coins of the era, and often depict a man with a strongly prominent nose and chin, and a heavy brow and forehead (Fig. 2).

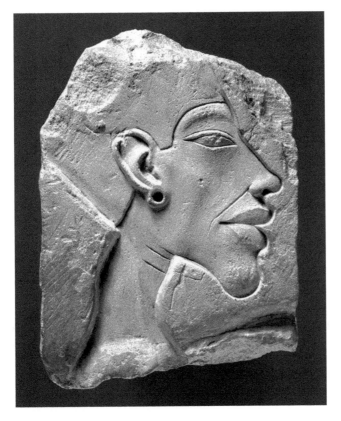

Figure 1
Portrait of Akhenaten, pharaoh of the 18th dynasty in Egypt. The profile of
Akhenaten as depicted here may be suggestive of acromegaly, particularly the
prominent nature of the mouth and lower jaw.
Source: Staatliche Museen zu Berlin—Preußischer Kulturbesitz, Ägyptisches Museum
Photo: Margarete Büsing

THE MIDDLE AGES AND THE RENAISSANCE

From what we know today of the epidemiology of acromegaly, it is likely
that pituitary adenomas have occurred at a relatively constant rate
throughout historical and present-day human populations. Our ancestors'
life spans were, however, significantly shorter than ours today, and many
individuals with growth hormone-secreting pituitary tumors probably
died of other causes before the telltale signs of the disease became apparent. For hard evidence of the existence of acromegaly, we must rely on the
archeological record of the Middle Ages. Hosovski (3) described the skeleton of a man from the 14th century excavated in Bosnia-Herzegovina,
whose skull demonstrated thickened supraorbital ridges, with prolonga-
tion of the mandible (Fig. 3). X-rays of the skull showed bony thickening

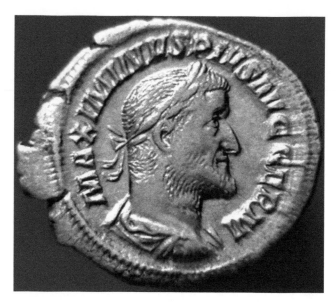

Figure 2
Portrait of the Roman Emperor Gaius Julius Verus Maximinus "Thrax" from a
sestersius of approximately 235 A.D. Maximinus Thrax was reputed to be a man of
gigantic stature who was capable of great feats of strength. Depictions of Maximinus
Thrax consistently portray him as having a prominent brow, nose, and jaw, which
have led some to suggest that he may have suffered from acro-gigantism.
Source: Adrian Daly
Photo: Vladimir Chichkov

and sinus enlargement, although the sella turcica was not grossly
abnormal. The rest of the skeleton showed extensive arthropathy and
marked osteophyte formation in the lumbar spine and coxarthrosis of
the right hip.

The first reliable medical description of acromegaly/gigantism
came from Johannes Wierus (Johann Weyer) in 1567 (Fig. 4). Wierus
was born in what is now The Netherlands, trained as a doctor in France,
and was an influential humanist writer who campaigned against the
persecution of the mentally ill as witches. For this work, Wierus has
been dubbed the "Father of Psychiatry." In his case collection *Medicarum
observationum rararum*, Wierus wrote about a female giant who made her
living by traveling and charging an entry fee to those who wished to see
her. The woman, whose parents were of normal height, developed
secondary amenorrhea at the age of about 14 and began to grow propor-
tionately and uniformly. When Wierus described her about 25 years
later, she was slow moving and had coarsened facial features, which
is suggestive of the effects of uncontrolled chronic growth hormone
hypersecretion.

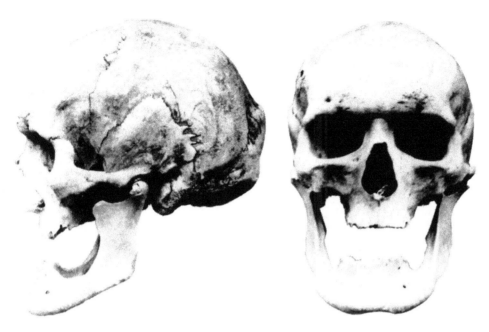

Figure 3
Photograph of the skull of a man from the 14th century excavated in
Bosnia-Herzegovina. The skull demonstrates prognathism and overgrowth
of the supraorbital ridges. Widespread bony thickening and arthroses were
present in the remaining bones of the skeleton. Radiography demonstrated
enlargement of the sinuses; however, the sella turcica was not grossly abnormal.
Source: From Ref. 3, with permission of E. Schweizerbart'sche Verlagsbuchhandlung (Naegele u.
Obermiller) Science Publishers, Stuttgart

LATE 18TH TO EARLY 20TH CENTURY: RECOGNITION AND DESCRIPTION OF ACROMEGALY

From the 18th through to the early 20th century, gigantism was popular-
ized as a medical curiosity and many persons were billed as the "world's
tallest," though few were measured accurately. For instance, beginning in
the mid-18th century, a series of giants from Ireland gained fame in Great
Britain and further afield. The first of these individuals was Cornelius
Magrath (1736–1760), who came to the attention of the general public in
1752, when he was 15 years old and measured over 7 feet 9 inches in
height. Thereafter, he traveled to England and then to continental Europe,
where he exhibited himself successfully during the 1750s. During travels
in Germany and Venice, Magrath was depicted artistically as is shown in
Figure 5. Unfortunately, this continuous touring, the poor care provided
by his managers, and his active disease contributed to rapidly failing
health. Magrath died after a fall at a theatre in 1760 at age 23. As was the
case with another Irish giant, Charles Byrne, the subject of a relentless

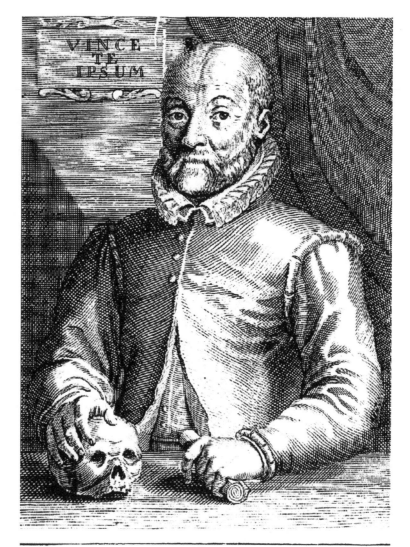

VINCE
TE
IPSUM

Joannes Wierus

Figure 4
Johannes Wierus (Johann Weyer), surgeon and humanist writer. In his
book *Medicarum observationum rararum*, published in 1567, Wierus included
what is probably the first medical description of a person with
acro-gigantism.
Source: United States National Library of Medicine

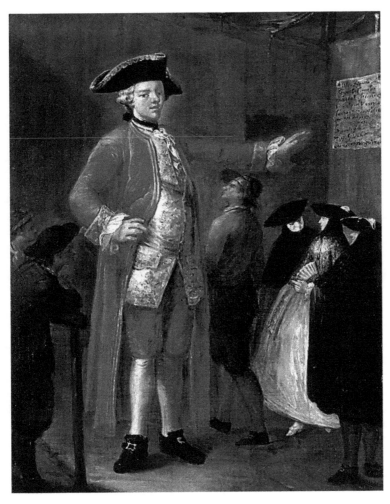

Figure 5
Portrait of the Irish Giant, Cornelius Magrath. This painting, entitled
"Il Gigante Magrat," was completed in 1757 by the artist Pietro Longhi
(1702–1785) while Magrath was visiting Venice as part of his exhibition
tour of Europe.
Source: Museo del Settecento Veneziano, Ca' Rezzonico, Venice, Italy
Photo: Cameraphoto Arte, Italy

pursuit by the anatomist John Hunter, Magrath's body became the topic of
a somewhat heated disagreement between Magrath's friends and anato-
mists and medical students. The latter group prevailed and a description
of the anatomical findings was delivered by Robert Robertson, the Professor of Anatomy at Trinity College, Dublin, in 1760. Magrath's skeleton is
preserved at the Department of Anatomy in Trinity College to this day. A
recent review of the gross pathology of Magrath's skeleton reveals marked

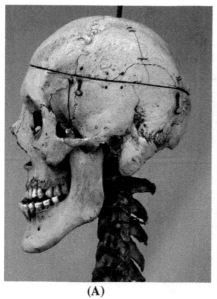
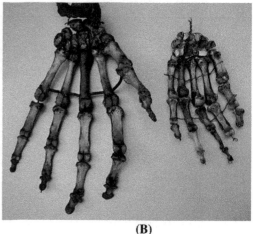

(A)   (B)

Figure 6
Acro-gigantic features of the skeleton of Cornelius Magrath. The skull (**A**)
demonstrates typical features of prognathism and overgrowth of the
supraorbital ridges, while the hand bones (**B**) are markedly lengthened in
comparison with the hand of a normal individual. In an engraving executed
for the purpose of publicity in Prussia, Germany in 1756, Magrath's middle finger
was said to be "as long as the hand of a full-grown man."
Source: Department of Anatomy, Trinity College, Dublin, Ireland
Photos: Paul Glacken

prognathism and other features of acromegaly/gigantism, as shown in
Figures 6 and 7.

   During the 19th century the popularity of touring spectacles, such as
circuses, increased further as a form of mass entertainment. Greater
enlightenment regarding the rights of performers and workers in general
also led to improved conditions for those "troupers" with gigantism that
toured individually or as part of shows. Indeed, the scientific interest in
the nature of acromegaly/gigantism was as intense as the popular interest
by the turn of the 20th century. For example, Fermin Arrudi (1870–1913)
(Fig. 8), who was 2.29 meters in height, traveled regularly from his remote
home high in the Spanish Pyrenees of Aragon to tour Europe, North
Africa, and North and South America. While his marriage in Paris in
1897 merited enormous press coverage (Fig. 9), Arrudi's schedule also
included hugely popular visits to medical schools in Munich and Vienna
during the mid-1890s (4). In contrast to the iniquities suffered by earlier
individuals such as Magrath and Byrne, Arrudi enjoyed fame and wealth

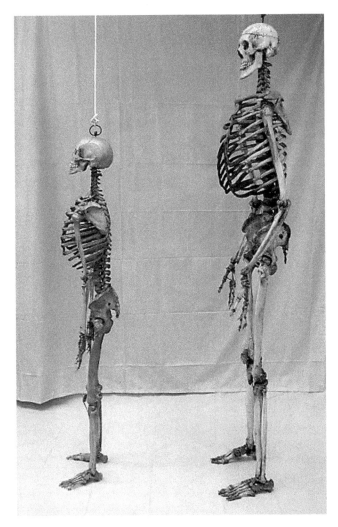

Figure 7
The skeleton of Cornelius Magrath. It has been estimated that Magrath stood between 7 feet 2 inches and 7 feet 9 inches (2.18 to 2.36 meters) in height when alive. The normal skeleton shown is approximately 5 feet 5 inches in height, which is close to the average height of his contemporaries of mid-18th century Europe.
Source: Department of Anatomy, Trinity College, Dublin, Ireland
Photo: Paul Glacken

and remained the master of his own affairs until he died, albeit at the early age of 43.

From the end of the 18th century onward, a series of landmark descriptions led inexorably to the recognition and naming of acromegaly as a distinct clinical entity by Pierre Marie in 1885. In 1772, Saucerotte reported to the French Academy of Surgery his description of notable

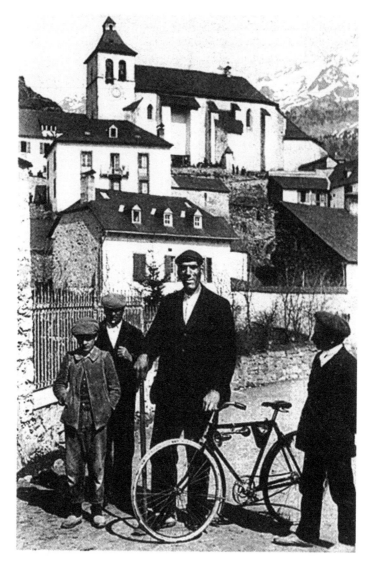

Figure 8
Photograph of the Spanish Giant, Fermin Arrudi (1870–1913). This photograph
was taken when Arrudi was in his 30s and demonstrates clear acromegalic
features. His height at the time was 2.29 meters. Note the use of a walking stick,
which Arrudi used frequently due to arthritis.
Source: Albert Beckers

bony overgrowth in a 39-year-old man, which was quite suggestive of
acromegaly and was later included in a compendium of presumptive
cases that established acromegaly as a distinct entity (5). Two early cases
describing the clinical and pathological features of acromegaly were published in Italy by Andrea Verga of Milan in 1864 (6) and by Vincenzo

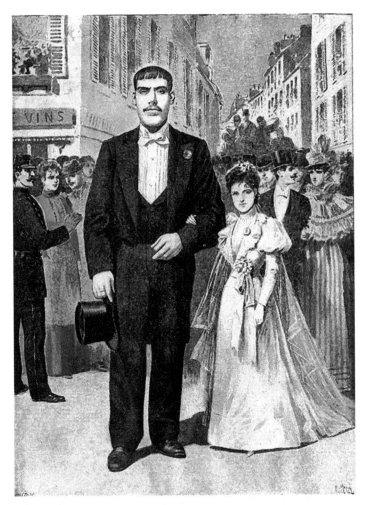

MARIAGE DE GÉANT

Figure 9
This illustration from the French periodical *Le Petit Journal* depicts Fermin Arrudi
and his wife Carla Dupuis following their wedding ceremony in Paris. Arrudi
traveled throughout Europe and the Americas at the turn of the 20th century and
was equally in demand with the medical profession as with the general public.
Arrudi was the subject of medical school lectures in Munich and Vienna about
the—as then—newly described disease of acromegaly.
Source: Wouter de Herder and Albert Beckers

Brigidi of Florence in 1881 (7). Verga's female patient had developed secondary amenorrhea at the age of 25 and gradual coarsening of her facial
features and changes in her body habitus were noted. In particular, she
reported having to have her rings readjusted repeatedly due to hand
enlargement. She also developed severe lower limb pain and visual

defects. The patient was hospitalized in 1856 and died in 1862 at age 59. At autopsy, Verga reported that the sella turcica was enlarged and that the pituitary had been replaced by a walnut-sized tumor compressing the optic chiasm. As noted by Brunori et al., while Verga's description of the potential disease mechanism was flawed, he pointed out correctly that early onset of the disease [which he termed prosopectasia, from *prosopon* (face) and *ektasis* (enlargement)] would lead to gigantism and that the visual defect was caused by tumor impingement on the optic nerves (8).

Brigidi's case was a popular Florentine actor called Ghirlenzoni, whose career was effectively ended by the progressive deformity and debilitation brought on by his disease. Ghirlenzoni committed suicide at age 65, and Brigidi, a pathologist, conducted an autopsy, during which he noted marked pituitary hypertrophy and skeletal changes typical of acromegaly. Probably the most significant finding was infiltration of the normal pituitary gland with cells of abnormal size and nuclear pattern.

Two Swiss doctors, Fritsche and Klebs, published an account in 1884 of the pathology of gigantism, which included a case report and illustrations of a man in his 40s who had been a longtime patient of Fritsche's (9). The illustrations very clearly show a man suffering from what we know now to be acromegaly, a finding that was reinforced by the finding of an enlarged pituitary on autopsy.

Pierre Marie, a neurologist working at the Salpétrière in Paris, first coined the term "acromegaly" in a paper submitted to *Revue de Medicine* in late 1885, which contained a description accompanied by photographs of two cases of patients with acromegaly (10). In this study, Marie noted acromegaly as being noncongential, distinct from other conditions like myxedema and Paget's disease, and typified by enlargement of the face and extremities. Subsequent publications in French and in English helped popularize the term acromegaly. One of these, in conjunction with Marie's Brazilian collaborator, de Souza-Leite, contained the first case collection of 48 possible cases of acromegaly (including Saucerotte's mentioned earlier) (5). Marie and de Souza-Leite also collected known autopsy results, noting the essential finding of pituitary and/or sellar enlargement.

By the late 1880s, a link had been made between the features of acromegaly and the finding of pituitary abnormalities on autopsy. However, it was not known how pituitary abnormalities actually produced acromegaly. Minkowski, describing a case of acromegaly in 1887 (11), did make the causal link between the pituitary tumor and acromegaly, but experimental evidence to back his claim was not available. In 1892, Massalongo (12), echoing the pathology report of Brigidi published 11 years earlier, noted the presence of microscopic abnormalities in the pituitary of a patient with acromegaly and suggested that this abnormality led to glandular hyperfunction. By 1900, histological methodologies had progressed sufficiently for Benda (13) to determine, in his series of normal and

diseased pituitaries, that acromegaly is associated with an eosinophilic
pituitary tumor.

LATE 19TH TO MID-20TH CENTURY: PATHOLOGY AND TREATMENT

As reported by Brunori et al. in their historical review, 1892 also saw the
publication by Vassale and Sacchi (14) of their experimental work on
transpalatal hypophysectomy in cats. They noted that complete pituitary
resection was invariably fatal, and by 1894 they felt confident enough of
their understanding of the pituitary to state "Its [the pituitary's] function
consists in the elaboration and endocrine secretion of a special product,
necessary to the body" (15). This work preceded by at least a decade the
canine hypophysectomy studies of Paulesco in Romania (16), whose
methodology was, in turn, adapted by Aschner in Vienna (17) and by
Harvey Cushing at Johns Hopkins in the United States (Fig. 10). The
work of both Aschner and Cushing during the first decade of the 20th
century provided the first hard experimental evidence of the role of the
anterior pituitary in the regulation of thyroid, gonadal, and metabolic
function and growth. These findings were presented by Cushing in a landmark paper published in the *Journal of the American Medical Association* in
1909, in which he summarized not only the structure and development
of the pituitary, but also introduced the terms "hyperpituitarism" and
"hypopituitarism" and described some of their clinical features including
acromegaly (18). As quoted by Medvei in *The History of Clinical Endocrinology* (19), Cushing also spoke of the role for which he is most famous,
namely that of neurosurgical pioneer, when he stated "When [symptoms
are] due to a tumor, surgery is the treatment that these conditions
demand."

Indeed, by that time (1909), neurosurgery for pituitary tumors was
an intensely active field, characterized by rapid advances and continuous
refinement. The first pituitary operation was attempted in the United
Kingdom by Caton and Paul in 1893, but unfortunately the tumor was
never reached successfully and the patient—who had acromegaly—did
not survive (20). Early results from a similar transcranial approach by
Horsley in ten patients between 1904 and 1906 were relatively poor,
although, as noted by Couldwell (21), Horsley's mortality rate of 20% con-
trasted favorably with the 50–80% mortality in patients operated upon by
his contemporaries. Schloffer reported the successful resection of a pituitary tumor via a transnasal transsphenoidal route in early 1907 (22) using
an approach developed by Giordano in cadaveric studies in 1897 (23).
This invasive operation required reflection of the entire nose to the right
via a deep incision from the glabella to the left nostril, and the subsequent
approach involved resection of the nasal septum and turbinates. The

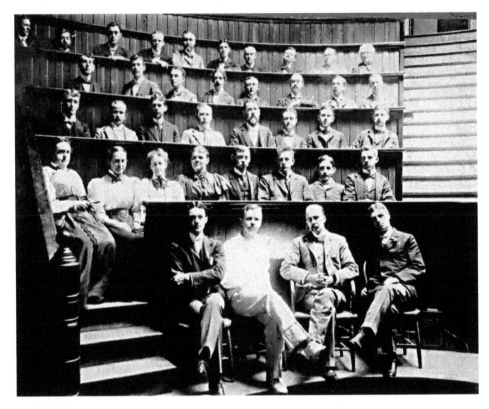

Figure 10
Graduating class and professors of the Johns Hopkins Medical School.
This undated photo taken between 1902 and 1912 shows Harvey
Cushing, then Associate Professor of Surgery (*front row, left*), alongside other
faculty members (*left to right*) Howard Kelly, Sir William Osler, and William
S. Thayer. Cushing was later to win a Pulitzer Prize for his biography of Osler.
Source: United States National Library of Medicine

Swiss surgeon Theodor Kocher improved on this technique in 1909 (24), in
the same year that he won the Nobel Prize for his work on thyroid disease. Kocher operated initially on an acromegalic patient and gained
access via a series of bilateral direct incisions through the nose, which
was followed by submucous dissection and preservation of the nasal
septum. At that time, Cushing had been using a transcranial approach to
the pituitary with poor results. In 1909, he performed his first transsphenoidal operation for acromegaly and used an adaptation of Schloffer's
technique (25). The 4th of June, 1910, saw the performance of two
operations, one by Oskar Hirsch in Vienna and the other by Cushing in
Baltimore, that augured the arrival of the modern surgical approach to
the pituitary used to this day. In Vienna, Hirsch, an otorhinolaryngologist,

pursued an endonasal, submucosal, transseptal, transsphenoidal approach to the pituitary under local anesthetic. Cushing used Halstead's suggestion of an initial sublabial incision followed by an adaptation of Kocher's technique, all under general anesthetic. As has been noted previously (26), while Cushing's approach represented a refinement of others' work, he scrupulously ascribed appropriate credit, particularly to Kocher and Halstead, under whom he had previously studied. Despite the utility, effectiveness, and good cosmesis afforded by the transsphenoidal approach, Cushing spent much of his career thereafter perfecting transcranial approaches. By the beginning of the 1930s, Cushing and the rest of U.S. neurosurgery had effectively discarded transsphenoidal approaches to pituitary adenomas.

The flame of transsphenoidal surgery was kept alive by a small number of neurosurgeons until it was repopularized in the 1960s. The aforementioned Oskar Hirsch had immigrated to Boston after the *Anschluss* brought Nazi rule to Austria in March 1938. At the Massachusetts General Hospital, he collaborated with the neurosurgeon Hannibal Hamelin; together, they commonly used the transsphenoidal route to reach the pituitary, effectively keeping the practice alive within the United States from the early 1940s until 1965 (27). Another key figure was Norman Dott, a Scottish neurosurgeon, who had trained on a Rockefeller fellowship with Cushing in Boston in 1923 before the latter had abandoned transsphenoidal pituitary surgery completely. Dott spent a large portion of his career perfecting his technique and introduced modifications that allowed greater illumination of the operative field. His surgical abilities were renowned, mortality rates were low due to his meticulousness, and, as has been suggested, his extensive pediatric surgical experience (27). These abilities and the continued utility of the transsphenoidal approach clearly impressed Gerard Guiot, the innovative French neurosurgeon, who learned the technique from Dott in 1956. Interestingly, Guiot was a pupil of Clovis Vincent, one of the founders of French neurosurgery who himself studied under Cushing in 1927. Guiot served as the axis around which the fortunes of transsphenoidal surgery changed among the neurosurgical community internationally. His introduction of radiological tools such as the fluoroscope and the image intensifier expanded the neurosurgeon's appreciation of the spatial relationships between instruments, tumor, and surrounding tissues within the small operative field. These improvements permitted more complete resection of difficult tumors while expanding the use of the technique to other tumor types.

The next significant advance in the development of the modern transsphenoidal technique came with the adaptation of the surgical microscope and televised fluoroscopy by Jules Hardy in Montreal, Canada (28). Microscopy and specially designed instruments permitted Hardy to identify more closely the borders of the normal and abnormal

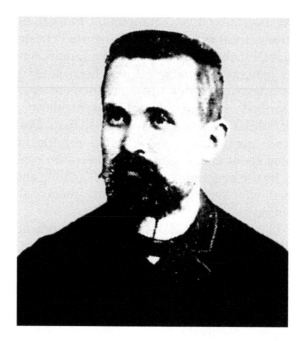

Figure 11
Antoine Béclère, French radiologist, who reported the first case of
radiotherapy of acromegaly in 1909.
Source: United States National Library of Medicine

pituitary tissues, thus aiding tumor resection while maximizing the
preservation of normal hypophyseal function. This experience with
microsurgery subsequently led to the fundamental reclassification of
pituitary tumors as micro- and macroadenomas.

Neurosurgery is not alone in having a distinguished history in the
treatment of hypophyseal disorders. The year 1909 saw not only the
publication of landmark pituitary surgical approaches by Kocher and
Cushing, but also the first use of radiotherapy for treating acromegaly
and gigantism. The French physician Béclère (Fig. 11) reported that some
local tumor-related symptoms (headache, visual disturbance) were
improved by repeated radiotherapy in a young female patient (29,30).
The same year, Gramagna reported another case of acromegaly treated
with radiotherapy (31). As noted by Lanzino and Laws (27), this approach
continued to be used during the early years of therapy for acromegaly,
with Oskar Hirsch applying radiation directly to the operative region as
a regular adjunct to surgery in order to reduce residual tumor size. Calculation of the required minimum effective radiation dose in pituitary tumor
treatment did not begin until the 1960s, after widespread use of mega-
voltage radiation equipment.

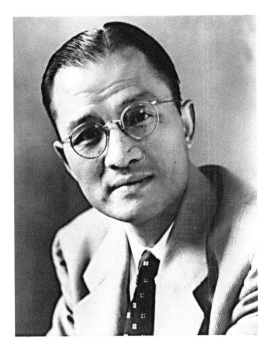

Figure 12
Choh Hao Li. While at the University of California, Berkeley, Li directed the
program that led to the isolation, purification, and characterization of pituitary
hormones such as growth hormone, follicle-stimulating hormone, luteinizing
hormone, and β-endorphin.
Source: United States National Library of Medicine

EARLY 20TH CENTURY TO PRESENT DAY: PHYSIOLOGY AND PHARMACOTHERAPY

In contrast to the pioneering spirit encountered during the first 25 years of
the 20th century, the subsequent history of pituitary endocrinology is one
characterized by gains in understanding that came at the cost of extraor-
dinarily laborious experimental methods. While thyroid hormone and
insulin were discovered at an early stage (1914 and 1921, respectively),
pituitary hormones were not isolated until the 1940s in a series of experiments led by the celebrated protein chemist Choh Hao Li (Fig. 12) at the
Berkeley, California, laboratory of Herbert Evans (Fig. 13). Over two
decades previously, Evans had provided the first experimental evidence
that pituitary hyperstimulation could cause an acromegaly-like syndrome
in rats (32). Li's painstaking work led to the isolation and determination of
molecular structure of not only growth hormone in 1945 (33), but also the
gonadotropins and adrenocorticotropic hormone in the 1940s and 1950s,
and β-endorphin in the late 1970s.

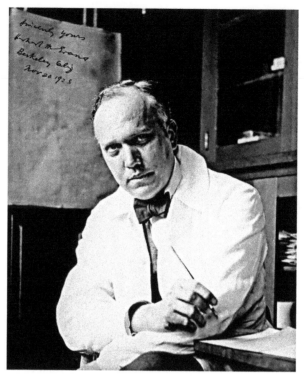

Figure 13

Herbert M. Evans, whose experimental work on the physiology of the
anterior pituitary during the 1920s and 1930s led to the development of
assays for pituitary hormones such as growth hormone. These studies,
summarized in his 1933 book, *The Growth and Gonad Stimulating Hormones
of the Anterior Hypophysis*, laid the groundwork for the studies of his collaborator
Li and others from the 1940s onward.
Source: United States National Library of Medicine

The research focus in the 1950s was expanding to encompass the
mechanisms by which pituitary hormonal secretion itself was governed.
The pivotal researcher of that era was Geoffrey Harris, who was largely
responsible for the formulation of the theory that the hypothalamus was
responsible for control of pituitary hormonal secretion via a series of
releasing or inhibitory factors. Harris was a prodigious and skilled experi-
mentalist and perfected the methods required to selectively ablate
hypothalamic and pituitary structure in rats and other small animals
without damaging surrounding structures. His studies, first at Cambridge
University and later at the Institute of Psychiatry at The Maudsley
Hospital, London, permitted the demonstration of hypothalamic–anterior
pituitary portal connections. Harris was hugely influential among young
endocrinology researchers at the time, and many assisted at his laboratory

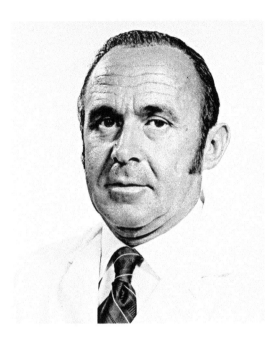

Figure 14
Andrew V. Schally. Awarded the Nobel Prize in 1977 for his contribution
to understanding the hypothalamic regulation of pituitary function, Schally
directed a highly focused program to isolate and characterize hypothalamic
hormones that relied on a combination of protein chemistry, physiology, and
industrial-sized processing of animal hypothalami.
Source: United States National Library of Medicine

learning his methods. The formulation of his theory that the hypothalamus controlled pituitary secretion via releasing factors that traveled via
the local portal vessels was a landmark step in endocrinology. However,
the validation of the theory represented an enormous challenge, as the
chemical nature of these still hypothetical factors was completely
unknown. The search for these hypothalamic factors led to a race of star-
tling intensity among at least four major research groups, led by Harris in
London, Samuel M. McCann in Pennsylvania and later Dallas, Andrew
Schally (Fig. 14) in New Orleans, and Roger Guillemin (Fig. 15) in Hous-
ton and later San Diego. As described by Nicholas Wade in his book *The
Nobel Duel* (34), both Harris's and McCann's teams were pursuing diverse
research projects during this period. Schally and Guillemin, however,
devoted their time single-mindedly to the identification of a series of
hypothalamic releasing factors. This research necessitated the collection
and processing of literally millions of animal hypothalami, often from
industrial sources, followed by purification, analysis, and testing by both
chemists and physiologists.

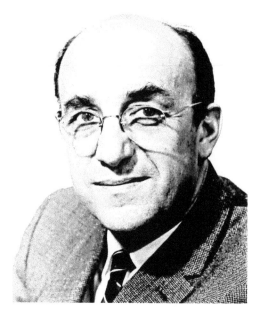

Figure 15
Roger Guillemin. Awarded the Nobel Prize in 1977 for his contribution
to understanding the hypothalamic regulation of pituitary function,
Guillemin directed groups in the United States and France that successfully
isolated important hypothalamic regulatory hormones such as
somatostatin.
Source: United States National Library of Medicine

From the late 1950s through to the early 1970s, the work of these rival
groups and associated colleagues was responsible for the identification of
the hypothalamic hormones that govern pituitary secretion, including
growth hormone releasing hormone and somatostatin. The systems used
at the time to measure hormonal activity were indirect bioassays, which,
in the case of growth hormone, measured the regeneration of epiphyseal
cartilage in young hypophysectomized rats (35). It came as a crucial
advance in the field when the radioimmunoassay was developed by
Berson and Yalow (Fig. 16). This permitted neuroendocrine researchers to
detect and measure accurately hormones secreted by the hypothalamic–
pituitary–peripheral gland axes. In recognition of this, Schally and
Guillemin were awarded the Nobel Prize in 1977 for their work contributing
to the discovery of the hypothalamic hormones (36,37)–an award that was
shared with Yalow for her development of the radioimmunoassay.

Despite the rapid acceptance of the radioimmunoassay in endocrinology, one of the most important discoveries regarding the physiology
of growth hormone was made on the basis of a discrepancy between

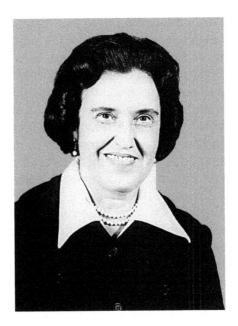

Figure 16
Rosalyn Yalow. Together with her collaborator, Solomon Berson, Yalow
was responsible for the development of the immunoassay, one of the
most important advances in medical research of the 20th century.
Radioimmunoassays revolutionized endocrinology by providing a reliable and
rapid method to measure hormone levels, even those present in vanishingly
small numbers. Yalow was awarded the Nobel Prize in 1977 in recognition
of the importance of this research.
Source: United States National Library of Medicine

the expected and observed results from bioassays. It had been noted in the
early 1950s that direct application of growth hormone to tissue cultures of
cartilaginous growth plates did not alter the rate of growth (35). In contrast, growth plates from animals treated systemically with growth hormone did exhibit enhanced growth despite the absence of growth
hormone from the tissue culture fluid (35). One such bioassay measured
the activity of growth hormone via the uptake of radiolabeled sulfate into
cartilaginous chondroitin sulfate. Salmon and Daughaday (38) demonstrated that sulfate uptake into cartilage from hypophysectomized rats
could not be influenced directly by growth hormone, but addition of serum
from normal rats or from growth hormone treated hypophysectomized
rats caused increased sulfate uptake. This idea of a circulating "sulfation
factor" that was induced by and mediated the effects of growth hormone
on peripheral tissues was termed the "somatomedin hypothesis" in the
1970s (39). The somatomedin that mediated growth hormone action was
designated as somatomedin-C, and by 1979 a radioimmunoassay for

somatomedin-C had been developed to assess disease activity in acromegaly (40). Another branch of research came at the problem from a different direction. Combining radioimmunoassay and bioassay techniques for insulin, Froesch et al. (41) had noted that a significant proportion of serum insulin-like activity was not suppressed by anti-insulin antibodies. Originally called "nonsuppressible insulin-like activity," it was eventually determined to be due to insulin-like growth factors (IGFs) I and II, and by the mid-1980s it had been shown that somatomedin-C and IGF-I were in reality one and the same (42,43). Circulating and locally produced IGF-I are now known to mediate growth signals across a wide variety of cells and tissues in health and disease (44).

Description of the various hypothalamic regulatory hormones also ushered in one of the principal therapeutic options for acromegaly available today, somatostatin analogs. Ladislav Krulich originally made the discovery of a hypothalamic factor that inhibited the secretion of growth hormone in 1968, while working as part of the McCann group (45). The following year, Hellman and Lernmark (46) described the inhibitory effects on insulin of a similar factor derived from the pancreas. Characterization of the polypeptide did not come until 1973, following the work of Paul Brazeau with Guillemin's group; it was they who termed the newly discovered hormone "somatostatin" (47). Collaborations between laboratories at pharmaceutical companies and academic groups were prominent during the discovery of hypothalamic regulatory hormones, particularly in the field of peptide chemistry. Following the characterization of somatostatin, a number of industry-based teams sought to develop long-acting somatostatin analogs, with the idea that such compounds could be useful in the treatment of diabetes mellitus. Initial studies with somatostatin in acromegaly did show a reduction in growth hormone secretion, but were limited by the short half-life of somatostatin (48). The discovery in the late 1970s that the activity of somatostatin could be reduced to a minimal amino acid sequence led to the development of the longer-acting octapeptide analog, octreotide, in 1982 (49). Understanding of the regulation of pituitary secretion of growth hormone and prolactin had progressed to the stage that dopaminergic pathways were being harnessed for the treatment of acromegaly by the mid-1970s (50).

CONCLUSION

By the 1980s, what we now view as the traditional treatments for acromegaly—surgery, radiotherapy, dopamine agonists, and somatostatin analogs—were available for use in patients. Since then, a great deal of study has been undertaken into the regulation of growth hormone axis activity, the genetics and pathology of pituitary tumors, the outcomes of treatment on morbidity and mortality in acromegaly, and the development of ever-stricter definitions of disease control. More recently still, molecular techniques have been used to determine the pathways by which growth is mediated at a cellular level. These techniques have provided both greater understanding of acromegaly and potent new therapeutic options.

REFERENCES

1. Starling EH. The Croonian Lectures on the chemical correlation of the functions of the body. Lecture I: The chemical control of the functions of the body. Lancet 1905; 2:339–341.

2. Sheaves R. A history of acromegaly. Pituitary 1999; 2:7–28.

3. Hosovski E. A case of acromegaly in the Middle Ages. Anthropol Anz 1991; 49(3):273–279.

4. Andolz Canela R. Fermin Arrudi. In: El Gigante Aragonés. Zaragoza: Mira Editores S.A., 1998.

5. Marie P, De Souza-Leite JD. Essays on Acromegaly. London: New Sydenham Society, 1891.

6. Verga A. Caso singolare di prosopectasia. Rend R 1 Limbardo Classe Sc Med Nat 1864; 1:111–117.

7. Brigidi V. Studii anatomo-patologici sopra un uomo divenuto stranamente deforme per cronica infermita. Arch Scuola Anat Patol Firenze 1881; 65–92.

8. Brunori A, Bruni P, Delitalia A, Chiapetta F. Acromegaly and pituitary tumors: early anatomoclinical observations. Surg Neurol 1995; 44:83–87.

9. Fritsche CF, Klebs TAE. Ein Beitrag zur Pathologie des Riesenwuchs. In: Klinische und pathologischananatomische Untersuchungen. Leipzig: Vogel, 1884.

10. Marie P. Sur deux cas d'acromegalie: hypertrophie singulére non congenitale des extrémitiés supérieures, inférieures et céphalique. Rev Med 1886; 6:297–333.

11. Minkowski O. Über einen Fall von Akromegalie. Berl Klin Wochensch 1887; 21:371–374.

12. Massalongo R. Sull'acromegalia. Rif Med 1892; 8:74–77.

13. Benda C. Beiträge zur normalen und pathologischen Histologie der menschlichen Hypophysis Cerebri. Klin Wochenschr 1900; 36:1205.

14. Vassale G, Sacchi E. Sulla distruzione della ghiandola pituitaria: richerche sperimentali. Riv Sper Freniatr Med Leg 1892; 18:525–561.

15. Vassale G, Sacchi E. Ulteriori esperienze sulla ghiandola pituitaria. Riv Sper Freniatr Med Leg 1894; 20:83–88.

16. Paulesco NC. L'hypophyse du cerveau. J Physiol Pathol Gen 1907; 9: 441–456.

17. Aschner B. Über die Funktion der Hypophyse. Pflügers Arch Physiol 1912; 146:1.

18. Cushing HW. The hypophysis cerebri: clinical aspects of hyperpituitarism and hypopituitarism. J Am Med Assoc 1909; 53:250–255.

19. Medvei VC. The History of Clinical Endocrinology. London: Parthenon, 1993.

20. Caton R, Paul FT. Notes of a case of acromegaly treated by operation. Br Med J 1893; 2:1421–1423.

21. Couldwell WT. Transsphenoidal and transcranial surgery for pituitary adenomas. J Neuro-Oncol 2004; 69:237–256.

22. Schloffer H. Erfolgreiche Operation eines Hypophysentumors auf nasalem Wege. Wien Klin Wochenschr 1907; 20:621–624.

23. Artico M, Pastore FS, Fraioli B, Giuffré R. The contributions of Davide Giordano (1864–1954) to pituitary surgery: the transglabellar–nasal approach. Neurosurgery 1998; 42:909–912.

24. Kocher T. Ein Fall von Hypophysis-tumor mit operativer Heilung. Dtsch Z Chir 1909; 100:13–37.

25. Cushing H. Partial hypophysectomy for acromegaly; with remarks on the function of the hypophysis. Ann Surg 1909; 50:1002–1017.

26. Liu JK, Das K, Weiss MH, Laws ER, Couldwell WT. The history and evolution of transsphenoidal surgery. J Neurosurg 2001; 95:1083–1096.

27. Lanzino G, Laws ER. Pioneers in the development of transsphenoidal surgery: Theodor Kocher, Oskar Hirsch, and Norman Dott. J Neurosurg 2001; 95:1097–1103.

28. Hardy J, Wigser SM. Trans-sphenoidal surgery of pituitary fossa tumors with televised radiofluoroscopic control. J Neurosurg 1965; 23:612–619.

29. Béclère A. Le traitment des tumeurs hypophysaires, du gigantisme et de l'acromegalie par la radio-thérapie. Bull Mem Soc Hôp Paris 1909; 27:274.

30. Béclère A. The radio-therapeutic treatment of tumours of the hypophysis, gigantism and acromegaly. Arch Roentgen Radiol 1909; 14:147.

31. Gramagna A. Un cas d'acromegalie traité par la radiothérapie. Rev Neurol 1909; 17:15.

32. Evans HM, Long JA. The effect of the anterior lobe of the pituitary administered intra-peritoneally upon growth, maturity and oestrus cycle of the rat. Anat Rec 1921; 21:62.

33. Li CH, Evans HM, Simpson ME. Isolation and properties of hypophyseal growth hormone. J Biol Chem 1945; 159:353–366.

34. Wade N. The Nobel Duel. Garden City, NY: Anchor Press-Doubleday, 1981.

35. Trueta J. Studies of the Development and Decay of the Human Frame. London: William Heinemann, 1968.

36. Schally AV. Aspects of hypothalamic regulation of the pituitary gland with major emphasis on its implications for the control of reproductive processes. Nobel Lecture, December 1977.

37. Guillemin R. Peptides in the brain. The new endocrinology of the neuron. Nobel Lecture, December 1977.

38. Salmon WD Jr, Daughaday WH. A hormonally controlled serum factor which stimulates sulfate incorporation by cartilage in vitro. J Lab Clin Med 1957; 49:825–836.

39. Daughaday WH, Hall K, Raben MS, Salmon WD Jr, van den Brande JL, Van Wyk JJ. Somatomedin: proposed designation for sulphation factor. Nature 1972; 235:107.

40. Clemmons DR, Van Wyk JJ, Ridgway EC, Kliman B, Kjellberg RN, Underwood LE. Evaluation of acromegaly by radioimmunoassay of somatomedin-C. N Engl J Med 1979; 301:1138–1142.

41. Froesch ER, Burgi H, Ramsier EB, Bally P, Labhart A. Antibody suppressible and nonsuppressible insulin-like activities in human serum and their physiologic significance. An insulin assay with adipose tissue of increased precision and specificity. J Clin Invest 1963; 42:1816–1834.

42. Klapper DG, Svoboda ME, Van Wyk JJ. Sequence analysis of somatomedin-C: confirmation of identity with insulin-like growth factor-I. Endocrinology 1983; 112:2215–2217.

43. Daughaday WH, Hall K, Salmon WD Jr, van den Brande JL, Van Wyk JJ. On the nomenclature of the somatomedins and insulin-like growth factors. J Clin Endocrinol Metab 1987; 65:1075–1076.

44. Le Roith D, Bondy C, Yakar S, Liu JL, Butler A. The somatomedin hypothesis. Endocr Rev 2001; 22:53–74.

45. Krulich L, Dhariwal AP, McCann SM. Stimulatory and inhibitory effects of purified hypothalamic extracts on growth hormone release from rat pituitary in vitro. Endocrinology 1968; 83:783–790.

46. Hellman B, Lernmark A. Inhibition of the in vitro secretion of insulin by an extract of pancreatic alpha-1 cells. Endocrinology 1969; 84:1484–1488.

47. Brazeau P, Vale W, Burgus R, Ling N, Butcher M, Rivier J, Guillemin R. Hypothalamic polypeptide that inhibits the secretion of immunoreactive pituitary growth hormone. Science 1973; 179:77–79.

48. Besser GM, Mortimer CH, Carr D, Schally AV, Coy DH, Evered D, Kastin AJ, Tunbridge WMG, Thorner MO, Hall R. Growth hormone release inhibiting hormone in acromegaly. Br Med J 1974; 1:352–355.

49. Bauer W, Briner U, Doepfner W, Haller R, Huguenin R, Marbach P, Petcher TJ, Pless J. SMS 201–995: a very potent and selective octapeptide analogue of somatostatin with prolonged action. Life Sci 1982; 31:1133–1140.

50. Wass JAH, Thorner MO, Morris DV, Rees LH, Mason SA, Jones AE, Besser GM. Long-term treatment of acromegaly with bromocriptine. Br Med J 1977; 1:875–878.

2

The Pituitary Gland:
Normal GH/IGF-I Secretion

ANATOMY AND STRUCTURE OF
THE PITUITARY GLAND

The pituitary gland comprises an anterior portion (adenohypophysis) and a posterior portion (neurohypophysis), each of which has a distinct embryonic origin. The adenohypophysis itself consists of three subdivisions, the pars distalis, the pars intermedia, and the pars tuberalis, all of which develop during embryonic life from Rathke's pouch, a region of the oral cavity. The posterior pituitary develops from the diencephalon as the median eminence, the neural stalk, and the posterior lobe. The final structure of the pituitary as anterior lobe (formed by the pars distalis), pituitary stalk (formed by the neural stalk and pars tuberalis), and posterior lobe begins to form during the second month of embryonic life. Differentiated glandular anterior lobe cells are detected during the second month of gestation, and all cell types are present by the end of the first trimester. Functional activity of the pituitary cells begins at the end of the second month of gestation; the final cell types to become functional, the mammotropes, become active at about the fifth month of intrauterine life.

The adult pituitary measures approximately 13 mm across by 6 mm high and is 9 mm in anteroposterior depth. In adults, the pituitary weighs from 0.5 to 1.0 g depending on age and sex; the pituitary is larger in younger individuals and in females. The pituitary sits in a region of the skull base called the hypophyseal fossa of the sella turcica ("Turkish saddle"). Inferolaterally, the pituitary is bounded by the sphenoid bone, below which lies the sphenoid sinus. The pituitary is covered superiorly by the diaphragma sellae, a section of dura through which the pituitary stalk passes to connect with the hypothalamus. Superior to the diaphragma sellae lies the optic chiasma. Laterally, the walls of the sella turcica are formed by the cavernous sinuses, which contain the internal carotid artery, and cranial nerves III, IV, V_1, V_2, and VI.

Histologically, the anterior pituitary consists of zones of glandular tissue of distinct secretory potential, which are invested with a rich sinusoidal network of blood vessels. Hormone-secreting anterior pituitary cells were previously classified according to their uptake of histological stains (acidophil, basophil, chromophobe); however, it is more informative to subdivide these cells according to the hormone(s) each produces.

The most common cell type is the *somatotroph*, which accounts for about half of the anterior lobe cells and is responsible for the production of the growth hormone (GH). Somatotrophs are mainly located in the lateral regions of the anterior lobe and are medium-sized, with a prominent intracellular secretory apparatus (Golgi and rough endoplasmic reticulum). The secretory granules in somatotrophs range in size from 150 nm to more than 800 nm in diameter. Larger granules are usually associated with the so-called somatomammotropes, a subset of cells that produce both GH and prolactin.

Lactotrophs/mammotrophs secrete prolactin and account for up to 25–30% of cells of the anterior lobe. They are located throughout the anterior lobe, with specific concentrations near the pars nervosa. Lactotrophs display a wide range of morphologies and ultrastructural features; these variations are most prominent during pregnancy and lactation when the cells may undergo marked hypertrophy.

Corticotrophs are thought to comprise about 10% of cells of the anterior lobe and are centrally located. Immunohistochemical analysis of these cells demonstrates positivity for pro-opiomelanocortin and its derivative peptides, adrenocorticotropic hormone (ACTH), β-endorphin, and β-lipotropin.

Gonadotrophs account for up to 20% of the cells of the anterior lobe and are located throughout the lobe. These cells can produce both luteinizing hormone (LH) and follicle stimulating hormone (FSH) or each hormone singly; they undergo variation in size according to sex hormonal status (i.e., gonadotrophs increase in size post-menopausally or following chemical or surgical castration).

Thyroid stimulating hormone (TSH)-immunoreactive *thyrotrophs* comprise about 5–10% of anterior lobe cells and are located in a relatively discrete anteromedial portion of the lobe. As is the case with lactotrophs and gonadotrophs, thyrotrophs can undergo impressive ultrastructural changes; in hypothyroidism, they undergo morphological changes of the rough endoplasmic reticulum and Golgi apparatus with protein accumulation.

The vascular supply of the anterior pituitary has been the subject of great historical debate and controversy over the years, particularly following the development of the theory of hypothalamic regulatory factor control of anterior pituitary function by Geoffrey Harris. The superior hypophyseal arteries supply the median eminence and part of the stalk before forming a superficial capillary plexus, which recoalesces to form long portal vessels that end in an internal plexus within the anterior lobe itself in close approximation to hormone-secreting cells. A series of short portal vessels also pass from the posterior into the anterior lobe and comprise about 25% of its blood supply. The majority of blood flow is from the hypothalamus to the pituitary, but there may be a short loop of pituitary feedback directly to the hypothalamus via the vessels derived from the middle hypophyseal artery. Blood (containing pituitary hormones) leaves the anterior pituitary via a venous system that empties into the systemic circulation via the internal jugular vein.

THE GROWTH HORMONE–INSULIN-LIKE GROWTH-FACTOR-I AXIS

Growth Hormone

Growth hormone (GH) is encoded by the *GH1* gene located on chromosome 17q22–q24, where it is found as part of a cluster that includes genes for placental lactogen and GH-V, or placental growth hormone (*GH2*). GH and placental lactogen (PL) are homologous proteins sharing about 85% of their amino acid sequences. GH and PL diverged functionally between about 40 and 60 million years ago; GH, PL, and prolactin all share a common ancestral genetic origin, with GH/PL diverging from prolactin about 400 million years ago (1). Mutations of the *GH1* gene or deletions of the surrounding regions can cause sporadic and inherited forms of growth deficiency and short stature (2,3).

GH is a 22 kDa protein of 191 amino acids that is derived from a 217-amino acid precursor molecule. The tertiary structure of the GH molecule is composed of four α-helices, and it has two disulfide bridges. A 20 kDa variant of GH is also encoded by *GH1* and arises as a splice variant (4). Larger dimeric ("big") and oligomeric ("big-big") forms of GH have been identified using electrophoresis, but probably do not have biological function (5). GH-V, placental GH, is the dominant form of GH circulating during pregnancy and is responsible for determining insulin-like growth factor-I (IGF-I) secretion (6,7).

GH mediates its actions via the GH receptor. GH binds to two receptor molecules and activates signaling. The signal transduction that follows GH receptor dimerization results in the activation of the protein kinase JAK2 which then tyrosine phosphorylates STAT5, a protein which can directly lead to activation of transcription of GH inducible genes (8). Approximately 40–50% of circulating GH is complexed to GH binding protein (GHBP) (9–11). GHBP has the same sequence as the extracellular domain of the GH receptor and is generated by specific proteolysis of the GH receptor. GHBP appears to protect circulating GH from degradation, thus increasing the half-life of GH (12).

GH mediates its growth-promoting effects both directly via the GH receptor and indirectly via the stimulation of IGF-I synthesis, particularly from the liver. GH receptor-mediated signaling stimulates growth and differentiation in tissues such as cartilage growth plates to induce longitudinal bone growth, and probably plays an important role in embryonic development. GH-induced IGF-I secretion is responsible for multiple proliferative and anti-apoptotic effects, promotes differentiation across most tissue types, and has a series of important metabolic functions.

Regulation of GH Secretion

In normal humans, GH secretion follows a pulsatile and diurnal pattern, with peaks of GH entering the circulation approximately every 2 to 4 h, predominately at night. Daytime levels in healthy adults should be very low or undetectable. Females secrete approximately 30% more GH than do males, and secretion rises in response to physical exercise and other physical stressors. Daily GH secretion in adults varies inversely with age; in adolescence, secretion and peak amplitude are greatly increased.

GH secretion is regulated by a series of hormonal and biochemical factors, and the interplay between these factors can be complex (Fig. 1). GH releasing hormone (GHRH) and somatostatin play important antagonistic roles in the secretion of GH, the former being a stimulator and the latter an inhibitor. GHRH is released by neurons in the median eminence and the infundibular nucleus of the hypothalamus while, locally, somatostatin is derived from the paraventricular nucleus. Pulsatile GHRH release from the hypothalamus is a powerful stimulator of preformed granular GH secretion from the pituitary. Other effects of GHRH include the stimulation of GH synthesis by somatotrophs and the stimulation of somatostatin secretion. In contrast, somatostatin inhibits the release of GH but not its synthesis and also appears to sensitize somatotrophs to subsequent GHRH stimulation. The overall effect of this balance between somatostatin and GHRH is to facilitate the burst release of GH in response to pulses of GHRH. In the hypothalamus, somatostatin acts to inhibit GHRH release. GH, in turn, stimulates IGF-I release from the liver and other tissues, and then feeds back to stimulate somatostatin and inhibit GHRH. The functioning of this regulatory network is further modulated

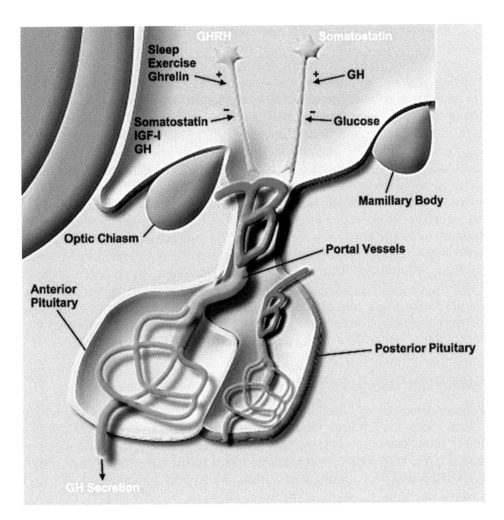

Figure 1

Hypothalamic regulation of growth hormone (GH) secretion. Secretion
of GH by the anterior pituitary is governed by a balance between inhibitory
and stimulatory signals. Somatostatin is a principal physiological regulator of
GH secretion and is itself modulated by GH and glucose. Hypothalamic GH
releasing hormone (GHRH) is the major physiological stimulator of GH
secretion by the pituitary; GHRH secretion is under the control of hormonal
factors, such as GH, IGF-I, somatostatin and ghrelin and physical factors
such as sleep and exercise.

Source: A. Beckers and P. Petrossians

by up- and down-regulation of somatostatin and GHRH receptor numbers and the actions of other hormones that dictate growth, particularly the sex steroids.

Another regulator of GH secretion is ghrelin, a relatively recently identified hormone that is secreted primarily by the stomach which has a host of important regulatory effects on pituitary and gastrointestinal function and energy metabolism. Ghrelin was discovered some time after its receptor had been identified as a means for modulating GH secretion using GH secretagogues. The nature of the role of ghrelin in GH regulation is still being determined, however, it mediates a significant effect on somatotroph GH secretion. The effect of ghrelin on GH release increases during adolescence, is maximal in adulthood, and then undergoes age-related decreases. In the hypothalamus, ghrelin appears to increase GHRH release. However, the mechanisms by which GHRH and ghrelin induce GH release from the pituitary appear to be different. Indeed, blockade of GH release via a GHRH antagonist was not associated with a change in circulating ghrelin levels (13). A modulatory role via somatostatin has also been suggested (14). Damage to hypothalamic structures appears to limit the action of ghrelin, thus supporting the hypothalamus as the major site of action of ghrelin in GH regulation (15). It may be that ghrelin is responsible for GH changes in response to fasting and food intake, rather than acting as a mediator of GH pulse production (14).

Insulin-Like Growth Factor-I

IGF-I is encoded by the *IGF1* gene on chromosome 12q22–q24.1, which has six exons and undergoes tissue-specific selective splicing (16,17). IGF-I is a 70-amino acid protein that contains three disulfide bridges and is 7.6 kDa in size. It is synthesized as a precursor protein and undergoes proteolysis of amino and carboxyl-terminal fragments. IGF-I and proinsulin probably share a common ancestor, but divergence occurred hundreds of millions of years ago (18). Mutations in the *IGF1* gene are associated with growth deficiency, deafness, and cognitive impairment. Polymorphisms in the *IGF1* gene govern variations in IGF-I levels in the general population, which may be linked, in turn, with altered risks of common diseases. For example, higher total IGF-I levels may be associated with an increased cancer risk, while lower IGF-I levels appear associated with an increased risk of cardiovascular disease (19–22).

The IGF system is highly complex and includes IGF-I and the related protein IGF-II, two receptors, IGFRI and IGFRII, six IGF binding proteins (IGFBP 1–6), a series of IGFBP-related proteins, and regulatory proteases. This network also interacts with other regulatory systems, and the expression of individual members of the IGF system is influenced by feedback events and gene expression regulatory events. The IGFBPs are themselves a superfamily of proteins that share important structural components (17).

They function to regulate circulating and tissue levels of IGF-I and IGF-II and modulate ligand receptor interactions. Indeed, the IGFBPs exhibit IGF-independent functions in their own right and are themselves regulated by a complex system of proteases (18).

IGF-I can act in a classical endocrine fashion and also in an autocrine or paracrine fashion at the local tissue level. "Endocrine" IGF-I is predominantly synthesized by the liver in response to pulses of pituitary GH. Thereafter, circulating IGF-I binds predominantly to IGFBP-3 and a second protein, acid-labile subunit, to form what is known as the 150 kDa complex. The regulation of IGF-I secretion by GH is subject to control by other hormones such as estrogen, prolactin, and thyroid hormones. Acting in a classically endocrine manner, IGF-I can mediate growth, as demonstrated by IGF-I infusions in experimental studies involving hypophysectomized animals (23–25). Endocrine IGF-I has an important role in the feedback control of pituitary GH secretion; increases in circulating IGF-I concentrations result in negative feedback and decreased GH release. Autocrine and paracrine actions of locally synthesized IGF-I are responsible for mediating a significant proportion of the other effects attributed to IGF-I. The range of cells thought to generate IGF-I in response to GH and subsequently grow includes chondrocytes, myocytes, and osteocytes. These local effects of IGF-I include modulation of differentiation, cell cycle control, regulation of cell survival (apoptosis), and various aspects of embryogenesis (26–33). Apart from growth, IGF-I plays an important role in regulating carbohydrate metabolism, predominantly via modulating insulin sensitivity (32). IGF-I and GH have opposite effects on insulin sensitivity, and IGF-I can decrease GH-related insulin resistance by feedback inhibition of GH secretion. IGF-I also has a direct insulin-sensitizing effect, probably via actions on the insulin receptor or related signaling molecules. Endocrine IGF-I levels appear to be more important than autocrine/paracrine IGF-I in the modulation of insulin sensitivity, while the latter may be more important in the regulation of growth.

REFERENCES

1. Owerbach D, Rutter WJ, Martial JA, Baxter JD, Shows TB. Genes for growth hormone, chorionic somatommammotropin, and growth hormone-like gene on chromosome 17 in humans. Science 1980; 209(4453):289–292.

2. Phillips JA III, Cogan JD. Genetic basis of endocrine disease. 6. Molecular basis of familial human growth hormone deficiency. J Clin Endocrinol Metab 1994; 78(1):11–16.

3. Millar DS, Lewis MD, Horan M, Newsway V, Easter TE, Gregory JW, Fryklund L, Norin M, Crowne EC, Davies SJ, Edwards P, Kirk J, Waldron K, Smith PJ, Phillips JA III, Scanlon MF, Krawczak M, Cooper DN, Procter AM. Novel mutations of the growth hormone 1 (GH1) gene disclosed by

modulation of the clinical selection criteria for individuals with short stature. Hum Mutat 2003; 21(4):424–440.

4. Masuda N, Watahiki M, Tanaka M, Yamakawa M, Shimizu K, Nagai J, Nakashima K. Molecular cloning of cDNA encoding 20 kDa variant human growth hormone and the alternative splicing mechanism. Biochim Biophys Acta 1988; 949(1):125–131.

5. Stolar MW, Baumann G, Vance ML, Thorner MO. Circulating growth hormone forms after stimulation of pituitary secretion with growth hormone-releasing factor in man. J Clin Endocrinol Metab 1984; 59(2):235–239.

6. Frankenne F, Rentier-Delrue F, Scippo ML, Martial J, Hennen G. Expression of the growth hormone variant gene in human placenta. J Clin Endocrinol Metab 1987; 64(3):635–637.

7. Beckers A, Stevenaert A, Foidart JM, Hennen G, Frankenne F. Placental and pituitary growth hormone secretion during pregnancy in acromegalic women. J Clin Endocrinol Metab 1990; 71(3):725–731.

8. Herrington J, Carter-Su C. Signaling pathways activated by the growth hormone receptor. Trends Endocrinol Metab 2001; 12(6):252–257.

9. Mannor DA, Winer LM, Shaw MA, Baumann G. Plasma growth hormone (GH)-binding proteins: effect on GH binding to receptors and GH action. J Clin Endocrinol Metab 1991; 73(1):30–34.

10. Baumann G, Mercado M. Growth hormone-binding proteins in plasma. Nutrition 1993; 9(6):546–553.

11. Baumann G. Growth hormone binding protein. The soluble growth hormone receptor. Minerva Endocrinol 2002; 27(4):265–276.

12. Amit T, Youdim MB, Hochberg Z. Clinical review 112: Does serum growth hormone (GH) binding protein reflect human GH receptor function? J Clin Endocrinol Metab 2000; 85(3):927–932.

13. Barkan AL, Dimaraki EV, Jessup SK, Symons KV, Ermolenko M, Jaffe CA. Ghrelin secretion in humans is sexually dimorphic, suppressed by somatostatin, and not affected by the ambient growth hormone levels. J Clin Endocrinol Metab 2003; 88(5):2180–2184.

14. van der Lely AJ, Tschop M, Heiman ML, Ghigo E. Biological, physiological, pathophysiological, and pharmacological aspects of ghrelin. Endocr Rev 2004; 25(3):426–457.

15. Popovic V, Miljic D, Micic D, Damjanovic S, Arvat E, Ghigo E, Dieguez C, Casanueva FF. Ghrelin main action on the regulation of growth hormone release is exerted at hypothalamic level. J Clin Endocrinol Metab 2003; 88(7):3450–3453.

16. Smith PJ, Spurrell EL, Coakley J, Hinds CJ, Ross RJ, Krainer AR, Chew SL. An exonic splicing enhancer in human IGF-I pre-mRNA mediates recognition of alternative exon 5 by the serine-arginine protein splicing factor-2/alternative splicing factor. Endocrinology 2002; 143(1):146–154.

17. Rotwein P, Pollock KM, Didier DK, Krivi GG. Organization and sequence of the human insulin-like growth factor I gene. Alternative RNA processing

produces two insulin-like growth factor I precursor peptides. J Biol Chem 1986; 261(11):4828–4832.

18. Rinderknecht E, Humbel RE. The amino acid sequence of human insulin-like growth factor I and its structural homology with proinsulin. J Biol Chem 1978; 253(8):2769–2776.

19. Schernhammer ES, Holly JM, Pollak MN, Hankinson SE. Circulating levels of insulin-like growth factors, their binding proteins, and breast cancer risk. Cancer Epidemiol Biomarkers Prev 2005; 14(3):699–704.

20. Skalkidou A, Petridou E, Papathom E, Salvanos H, Chrousos G, Trichopoulos D. Birth size and neonatal levels of major components of the IGF system: implications for later risk of cancer. J Pediatr Endocrinol Metab 2002; 15(9):1479–1486.

21. Janssen JA, Lamberts SW. IGF-I and longevity. Horm Res 2004; 62(suppl 3):104–109.

22. Kaplan RC, Strickler HD, Rohan TE, Muzumdar R, Brown DL. Insulin-like growth factors and coronary heart disease. Cardiol Rev 2005; 13(1):35–39.

23. Russell SM, Spencer EM. Local injections of human or rat growth hormone or of purified human somatomedin-C stimulate unilateral tibial epiphyseal growth in hypophysectomized rats. Endocrinology 1985; 116(6):2563–2567.

24. Schoenle E, Zapf J, Hauri C, Steiner T, Froesch ER. Comparison of in vivo effects of insulin-like growth factors I and II and of growth hormone in hypophysectomized rats. Acta Endocrinol (Copenh) 1985; 108(2):167–174.

25. Zapf J, Schoenle E, Froesch ER. In vivo effects of the insulin-like growth factors (IGFs) in the hypophysectomized rat: comparison with human growth hormone and the possible role of the specific IGF carrier proteins. Ciba Found Symp 1985; 116:169–187.

26. Le Roith D, Bondy C, Yakar S, Liu JL, Butler A. The somatomedin hypothesis: 2001. Endocr Rev 2001; 22(1):53–74.

27. Cohick WS, Clemmons DR. The insulin-like growth factors. Annu Rev Physiol 1993; 55:131–153.

28. Rubin R, Baserga R. Insulin-like growth factor-I receptor. Its role in cell proliferation, apoptosis, and tumorigenicity. Lab Invest 1995; 73(3):311–331.

29. Bondy CA, Cheng CM. Signaling by insulin-like growth factor 1 in brain. Eur J Pharmacol 2004; 19:490(1–3):25–31.

30. Delafontaine P, Song YH, Li Y. Expression, regulation, and function of IGF-1, IGF-1R, and IGF-1 binding proteins in blood vessels. Arterioscler Thromb Vasc Biol 2004; 24(3):435–444.

31. Fowden AL. The insulin-like growth factors and feto-placental growth. Placenta 2003; 24(8–9):803–812.

32. Firth SM, Baxter RC. Cellular actions of the insulin-like growth factor binding proteins. Endocr Rev 2002; 23(6):824–854.

33. Edmondson SR, Thumiger SP, Werther GA, Wraight CJ. Epidermal homeostasis: the role of the growth hormone and insulin-like growth factor systems. Endocr Rev 2003; 24(6):737–764.

3

Epidemiology, Pathology, and Complications of Acromegaly

EPIDEMIOLOGY

The epidemiology of acromegaly has been described in a series of studies performed in different countries. Taking only those performed in the modern era, the incidence and prevalence figures for acromegaly are relatively constant (1–6). The first study of this era was performed in 1980 in Newcastle, United Kingdom and described patients diagnosed after 1971 (5). The reported incidence and prevalence rates are some of the lowest in the series at 2.8 cases per million population per year and 38 cases per million, respectively. Subsequent studies by Bengtsson in Gothenburg, Sweden (incidence 3.3 per million per year; prevalence 69 per million), Ritchie in Northern Ireland (incidence 4.0 per million per year; prevalence 63 per million), and Etxabe in the Basque Country, Spain (incidence 3.1 per million per year; prevalence 60 per million) have all reported consistently higher frequencies of acromegaly (2–4). The most recent data come from the Spanish Acromegaly Registry, which reported an incidence of 2.1 cases per million per year and a mean prevalence of 36 cases per million population, although the variation in prevalence was very large, from 15.7 to 75.8 cases per million (6). Taking these results together, it can be estimated that the average incidence of acromegaly is 3.06 cases per million population per year and the prevalence is 53.2 cases per million population.

As acromegaly is an insidious disease, there is commonly a delay between the time the first symptoms are noted and when the diagnosis is made. Reviewing the available literature, Holdaway and Rajasoorya (1) estimated that the delay in diagnosis of acromegaly ranged from 6.6 to 10.2 years, with an average delay of 8 years. In one study by Nabarro (7), it was reported that the delay before diagnosis in patients aged more than 50 years was over twice that in patients aged less than 30 years (12.3 and 6.0 years, respectively). The incidence rates in males and females are equal and the average age at diagnosis ranges from 40 to 50 years (1–4,6).

MORTALITY

With its high rates of associated morbidities, acromegaly carries an increased mortality risk compared to the general population. This increased mortality risk has been estimated as being between two and four times that of the general population (8,9). The major causes of mortality are cardiovascular disease and respiratory disease; cancer is an important cause of mortality in acromegaly, however, data supporting an increased risk of cancer in acromegaly are not entirely clear-cut. Table 1 shows data from studies in the literature reporting the causes of death in patients with acromegaly according to these three major headings. Across these studies, the average percentages of deaths attributed to cardiovascular disease, cancer, and respiratory disease were 47.3%, 26.4%, and 8.3%, respectively.

Table 1
Major Causes of Mortality in Acromegaly

Study (Ref.)	Cause of death(%)		
	Vascular	Respiratory	Cancer
Wright et al. (10)	38.5	18	18
Alexander et al. (5)	60	15.5	15.5
Nabarro (7)	55	6	23
Bengtsson et al. (4)	52	–	24
Bates et al. (8)	57	25	11
Etxabe et al. (2)	30	–	50
Rajasoorya et al. (9)	62.5	–	9
Swearingen et al. (11)	42	8	33
Beauregard et al. (12)	28	–	50
Arita et al. (13)	45.5	18	18
Ayuk et al. (14)	58	14	22
Holdaway et al. (15)	61	3	24
Biermasz et al. (16)	25	–	46

A series of predictors of poor outcomes in acromegaly have been identified, many of which are also predictors of a poor response to therapy. As reviewed by Holdaway and Rajasoorya, these prognostic factors can be divided into those that predict morbidity and those that predict mortality (1). Factors that are predictive of morbidity include large tumor size, suprasellar extension, a high preoperative growth hormone (GH) concentration, the last post-treatment GH level, and the duration of disease before diagnosis. Mortality predictors in acromegaly include hypertension, diabetes mellitus, the last post-treatment GH level, the duration from disease onset to diagnosis, and the age of the patient. Both mortality and morbidity were predicted to some extent by the extent of exposure to elevated GH. This review comprised many studies that were performed before the advent of standardized insulin-like growth factor-I (IGF-I) assays.

One of the most important advances to have occurred in the study of acromegaly during the last decade has been the demonstration of the impact of treatment on lowering mortality rates. An initial study by Bates et al. (8) demonstrated that acromegalic patients did not exhibit a mortality rate that was different from the general population if their nadir mean GH was $< 2.5\,\mu g/L$. Since then, multiple large studies performed at single centers have confirmed that when GH or IGF-I levels are controlled, mortality in acromegalic patients returns to that seen in the general population (11,15,16). For example, Holdaway et al. (15) in Auckland, New Zealand, reported that serum IGF-I was significantly associated with mortality, with an observed/expected mortality ratio of 3.5 for patients who had a standard deviation score for IGF-I of greater than 2. In groups with lower IGF-I standard deviation scores, mortality decreased in parallel to within the expected range for the general population. Similar data were shown for GH in this series. Other groups in the United States (11) and the Netherlands (16) have also shown that strict GH or IGF-I control in acromegaly is associated with normalized life expectancy. Taken together, these data form a compelling argument for striving to control excess IGF-I and GH secretion in all acromegalic patients.

PATHOLOGY: HISTOPATHOLOGICAL CHARACTERISTICS OF TUMORS IN ACROMEGALY

A variety of classification systems have been used to subdivide pituitary tumors according to histological staining, ultrastructural and immunochemical features, and pathological behavior/aggressiveness (17–20). Figures 1 and 2 demonstrate the histological differences in structure between adenomatous tissue and normal pituitary.

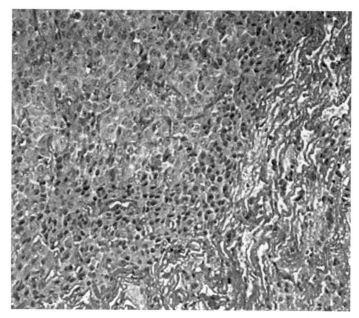

Figure 1
Histological section of a GH-secreting pituitary adenoma showing the border
between adenomatous tissue (*left*) and normal pituitary (*right*).
(PAS orange stain)
Source: J. Trouillas

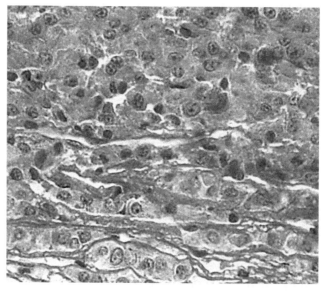

Figure 2
High-power magnification of the border zone separating a GH-secreting
pituitary adenoma from surrounding normal pituitary tissue.
(PAS orange stain)
Source: J. Trouillas

One of the more frequent subclassifications of GH-secreting pituitary tumors divides tumors by intracellular granule number into densely granulated and sparsely granulated adenomas (Figs. 3–6). These two morphological types differ in their clinical behavior, with sparsely granulated tumors more likely to be macroadenomas, to have a higher rate of extension and/or invasiveness, and to have poorer responses to somatostatin analogs (21). Cytokeratin patterns also appear to correlate with granularity and clinical behavior; the more responsive, densely granular tumors having perinuclear cytokeratin staining, while sparsely granulated adenomas are more aggressive and have a dotlike cytokeratin pattern (Fig. 7) (21,22).

Immunostaining techniques, such as staining for GH using an anti-GH antibody technique, as shown in Figures 8 and 9, can reveal positivity for hormones within resected tumor tissue. Electron micrograph views using double-gold immunostaining have been used to show the patterns of hormone expression in GH-secreting tissues, which can co-secrete prolactin in some cases (Figs. 10–13).

The effect of chronic pituitary stimulation by an ectopic GHRH-secreting tumor is shown in Figure 14, while histological positivity for GHRH is shown in a lung carcinoid (Fig. 15).

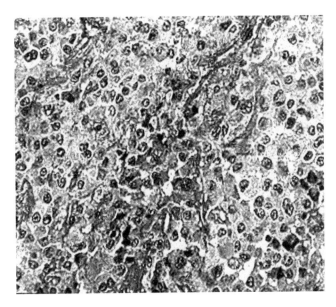

Figure 3
A densely granulated GH-secreting pituitary adenoma. GH-containing granules appear orange in color.
(Herlant tetrachrome stain)
Source: J. Trouillas

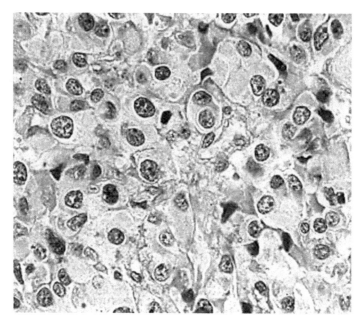

Figure 4
A sparsely granulated GH-secreting pituitary adenoma showing two cells containing orange-staining GH.
(Herlant tetrachrome stain)
Source: J. Trouillas

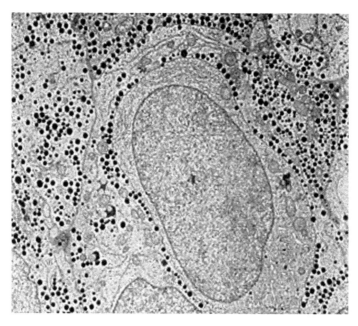

Figure 5
Electron micrograph of a densely granulated GH-secreting cell.
(GH-containing granules shown in black.)
Source: J. Trouillas

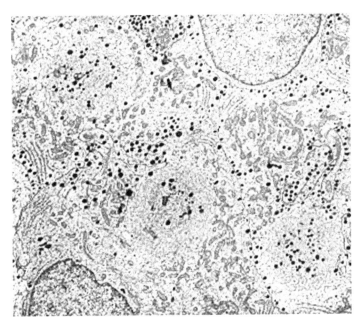

Figure 6
Electron micrograph of a sparsely granulated GH-secreting cell. Contrast the
low number of black GH-containing granules with the denser granulation
shown in Figure 5.
Source: J. Trouillas

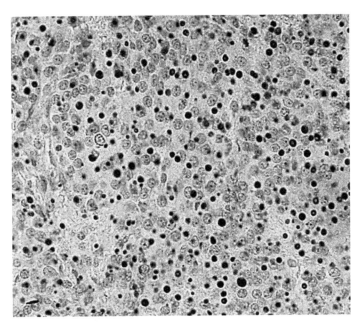

Figure 7
Cytokeratin staining in a sparsely-granulated GH-secreting adenoma.
(Anti-cytokeratin antibody stain)
Source: J. Trouillas

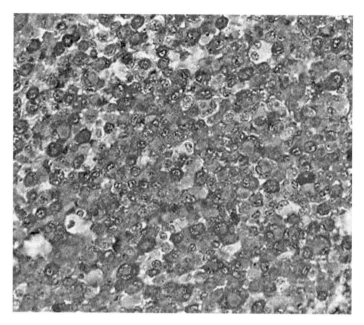

Figure 8
Anti-GH antibody immunostain of a GH-secreting pituitary adenoma showing
widespread positivity for GH (brown).
Source: J. Trouillas

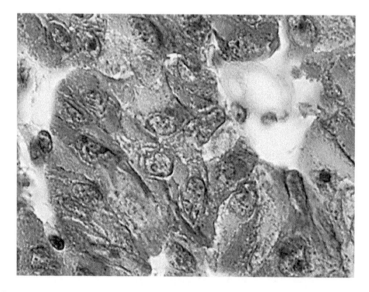

Figure 9
Strong immunostaining for GH in a section of GH-secreting pituitary adenoma
resected from a patient with acromegaly.
Source: J. Trouillas

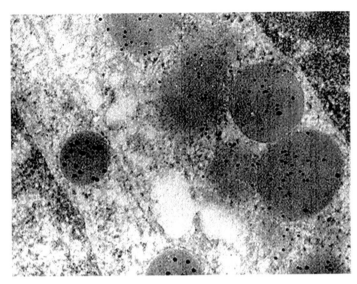

Figure 10
Electron micrograph showing double-gold immunocytochemical staining
of secretory granules containing GH (*left*) and other prolactin-positive
granules (*right*).
Source: A. Beckers

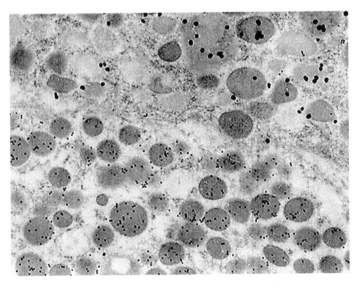

Figure 11
Electron micrograph showing double-gold immunocytochemical staining for
GH (smaller, 15 nm particles) and prolactin (larger, 40 nm particles).
Source: A. Beckers

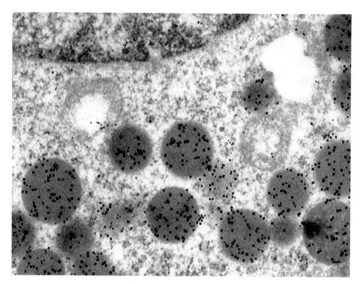

Figure 12
Electron micrograph of somatomammotroph cells stained simultaneously for GH
(15 nm particles) and prolactin (10 nm particles). Both hormones are present in
the same granules.
Source: A. Beckers

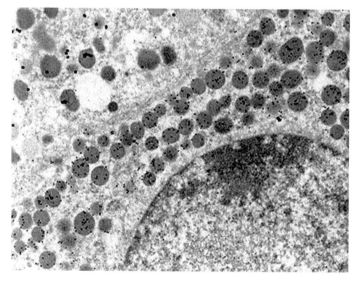

Figure 13
Electron micrograph showing double-gold immunostain in a mixed
GH/prolactin-secreting pituitary adenoma. A prolactin-secreting cell
is shown on the left, while a GH-secreting cell is on the right.
Source: A. Beckers

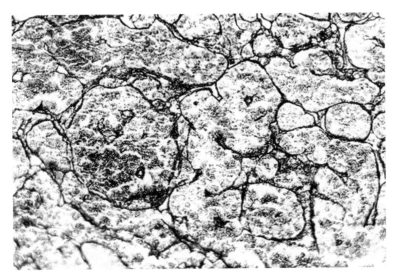

Figure 14
Pituitary hyperplasia due to the effects of a GHRH-secreting carcinoid tumor associated with GH hypersecretion and acromegaly. Gordon–Sweet silver stain shows preserved reticulin fiber network in the hyperplastic tissue.
Source: K. Kovacs and A. Beckers

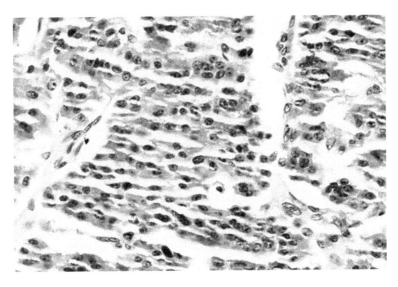

Figure 15
Immunostain showing GHRH positivity in a GHRH-secreting bronchial carcinoid tumor.
Source: K. Kovacs and A. Beckers

CAUSES OF ACROMEGALY

More than 95% of cases of acromegaly occur sporadically due to a pituitary adenoma in patients without genetic disease traits that are associated with endocrine tumors. Approximately 1% of cases are caused by such familial or inherited endocrine diseases as multiple endocrine neoplasia type I (MEN-1). Pituitary carcinomas are very rare and only 140 of any type have been reported in the literature; GH-secreting pituitary carcinomas are usually hormonally active and can behave as invasive adenomas until they metastasize, or they may metastasize early (23).

The remaining cases of acromegaly are due to GHRH hypersecretion from a site in the hypothalamus or ectopically that can induce pituitary hyperplasia; occasionally, GH secretion from ectopic pituitary tissue or an extra-pituitary tumor may induce acromegaly. Studies of the characteristics of patients with sporadic disease and the genetic and molecular profiles of their tumors have revealed some interesting potential causative factors, although none of these is definitive.

Sporadic Acromegaly

A variety of putative stimuli for pituitary adenoma formation have been suggested (20,24).

Hormonal hypersecretion. Hypothalamic GHRH hypersecretion has been shown to induce proliferation and hyperplasia of pituitary somatotroph cells and can induce pituitary adenoma formation.

Oncogenes. A mutated form of *gsp*, which encodes a constitutively active form of the G-protein, Gs_α, has been described in up to 40% of GH-secreting pituitary adenomas. In one study, patients with *gsp*-positive tumors had greater inhibition of GH by a somatostatin analog compared to patients without the *gsp* oncogene mutation (25). See also the discussion of McCune–Albright syndrome, which follows later in this chapter.

Other molecular and genetic factors. A series of newly identified factors, such as a pituitary derived truncated form of the fibroblast growth factor receptor-4 (ptd-FGFR4) and a pituitary tumor transforming gene (PTTG) product, have been suggested as modulators or stimulators of pituitary tumorigenesis (26–31). Loss of heterozygosity for regions of chromosome 11, including the *MEN1* gene locus, has been reported in some somatotropinomas (32) but not in others (33,34).

Inherited and Familial Acromegaly

MEN-1

MEN-1 is an autosomal dominant disease that is associated with endocrine tumors of the parathyroid and pancreas/gut, and anterior pituitary tumors (35). *MEN1*, the gene responsible for MEN-1 on chromosome 11q13, encodes the protein menin, which has a diverse range of regulatory actions (35). The phenotypic expression of MEN-1 can be caused by a wide range of genetic mutations that alter the structure or function of menin. In larger series, acromegaly occurs in up to 10% of cases of MEN-1 (36). The features of acromegaly in MEN-1 differ somewhat from those of sporadic acromegaly, with a greater female preponderance. Approximately 50% of MEN-1-related acromegaly is controlled by multi-modal therapy (surgery, medical therapy, radiotherapy).

Carney Complex

The Carney complex was originally described as an association of spotty skin pigmentation, myxomas, endocrine hypersecretion, and schwanno-mas (37). This rare condition is familial in 70% of cases and is due to muta-tions in the Iα regulatory subunit of protein kinase A type I (*PRKAR1A*) on chromosome 17q22–24, although another locus on chromosome 2p16 has also been implicated (38). As in MEN-1, mutations of the *PRKAR1A* gene are not associated with sporadic pituitary adenomas (39). In Carney com-plex, acromegaly occurs due to multifocal hyperplasia of somatomammo-tropic cells in the pituitary that eventually can form regions of GH/prolactin-secreting adenomatous tissue. The majority of patients (75%) with Carney complex have asymptomatic increases in GH, IGF-I, and prolactin or have abnormal dynamic pituitary test function.

McCune–Albright Syndrome

McCune–Albright syndrome is a complex of polyostotic fibrous dyspla-sia, café-au-lait skin pigmentation, and endocrine abnormalities, includ-ing precocious puberty, GH hypersecretion, and acromegaly (40). It is caused by mosaicism for a mutation of the gene *GNAS1* located on chromosome 20q13.2. One of the mutations associated with McCune–Albright syndrome is due to a single nucleotide substitution that changes the codon from that for arginine (Fig. 16) to that of cysteine (Fig. 17) at position 201 in the Gs_α molecule, which results in constitutional activation of the molecule. Approximately 20% of patients with this syndrome have disorders of GH excess, and in one-third of these, a pitui-tary adenoma is identifiable (40). The growth effects of combined GH and other hormonal hypersecretion, in addition to bony overgrowth, can lead to quite marked physical deformities in patients, as depicted in Figures 18 and 19.

Isolated Familial Acromegaly

A syndrome of isolated familial acromegaly is defined as two or more cases of acromegaly or gigantism in a family in the absence of MEN-1

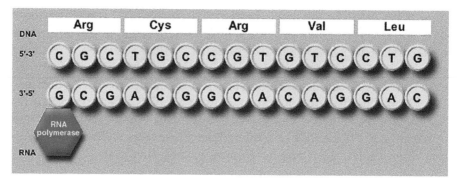

Figure 16
Normal genetic sequence of the *GNAS1* gene, which codes for arginine, cystine, arginine, valine, and leucine between positions 199 and 203.
Source: A. Beckers and P. Petrossians

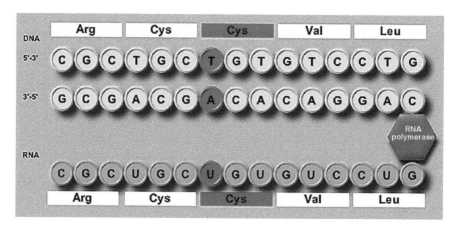

Figure 17
A mutation in the gene encoding Gs$_{\alpha}$ in McCune–Albright syndrome. A single C to T modification changes arginine at position 201 to a cysteine, leading to abnormal G-protein activation.
Source: A. Beckers and P. Petrossians

or Carney complex (41,42). Soares and Frohman (41) have recently calculated that more than 100 cases of isolated familial acromegaly or gigantism have been reported among 44 families in the literature. Acromegaly in this familial form appears to differ from sporadic acromegaly, with a younger age at diagnosis (25 years), a male-to-female ratio of 1.5:1, and an almost invariable presentation with macroadenoma. Linkage to chromosome 11q13 close to the *MEN1* locus has been suggested, but MEN-1 mutations are absent (41–44).

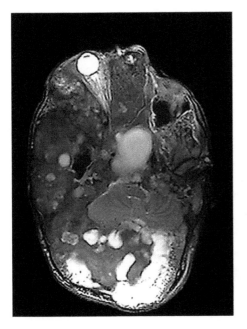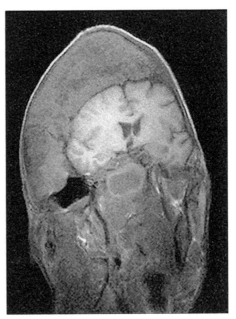

Figure 18
MRI images of the head of a patient with advanced McCune–Albright syndrome demonstrating deformities and compression of soft tissues due to bone overgrowth.
Source: A. Beckers and P. Petrossians

Ectopic Acromegaly

In a small number of cases, acromegaly may be caused by GHRH or GH hypersecretion from an ectopic endocrine-active tumor, such as a bronchial, gut, or thymic carcinoid (45–49). Some ectopic tumors may be located relatively close to normal pituitary tissue, for example in the sphenoid or cavernous sinus (50–52). Such tumors may express high concentrations of somatostatin receptor subtype 2, which can help in tumor localization and planning for surgery. Hypothalamic overproduction of GHRH has also been associated with acromegaly in rare cases, and may be due to the effects of a gangliocytoma (53).

GH Overtreatment and Abuse

It has been recognized recently that acromegaly symptoms, such as edema, headache, and arthralgias, can occur in GH-deficient patients taking GH replacement therapy at too high a dose (54). For hypopituitary patients receiving GH supplementation, serum IGF-I levels should be monitored closely and maintained within age-appropriate ranges. The indiscriminate use of GH as part of doping in sports has been acknowledged for some time (55,56) and may be a growing problem (57). GH

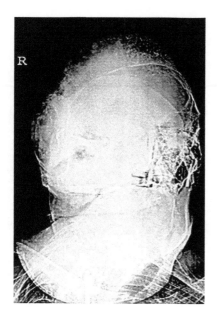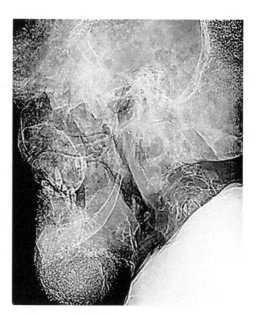

Figure 19
Plain skull radiographs of the head of the patient shown in Figure 18,
demonstrating clearly the effects of fibrous dysplasia and bony deformity
on the skull and mandible.
Source: A. Beckers and P. Petrossians

abuse has the potential to cause acromegaly in those taking excessive
doses over a period of years.

COMPLICATIONS OF ACROMEGALY

Acromegaly is associated with a wide range of pathological effects on
nearly all tissues and organs. The complications of acromegaly can be
caused by the direct expansion of a tumor, such as optic chiasmal impingement and visual field loss due to suprasellar extension of a macroadenoma (Fig. 20). The insidious effects of GH/IGF-I hypersecretion
are considerable, such that even the less harmful sequelae, like skin
thickening, actually represent profound architectural remodeling
(Figs. 21 and 22).
    As has been outlined previously, hormonal hypersecretion has a
negative impact on mortality via increased rates of deaths due to cardiovascular disease, respiratory disease, and, in some series, cancer. In parallel with our improved appreciation of how important hormonal control is
for the normalization of mortality rates, there has been an increased interest in diagnosing and treating the major complications of acromegaly.
Recent guidelines have provided a useful framework in which to consider

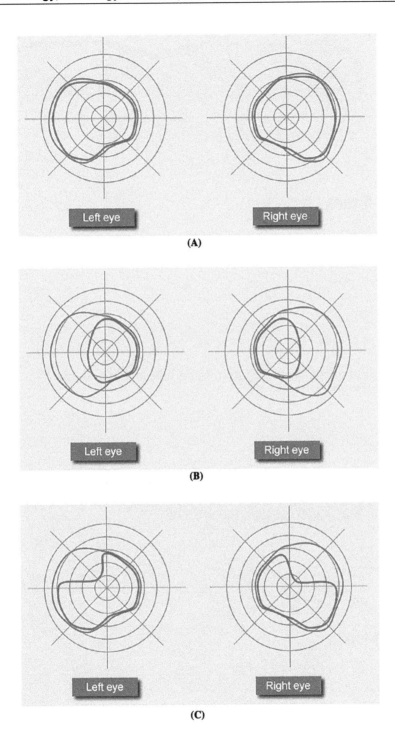

(A)

(B)

(C)

Figure 20

Possible visual field defects in acromegaly (blue outline: expected field; red outline: limited field). (**A**) Normal visual fields; (**B**) bitemporal hemianopsia; (**C**) temporal quadrantanopsias.

Source: A. Beckers and P. Petrossians

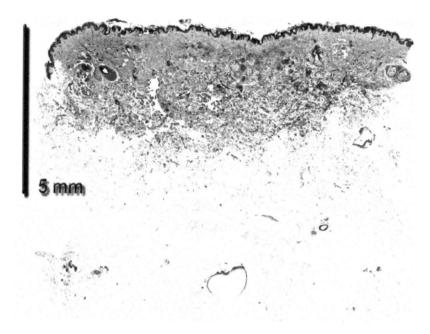

Figure 21
Skin biopsy showing normal epidermis, dermis, and hypodermis.
Source: A. Beckers and G. Piérard

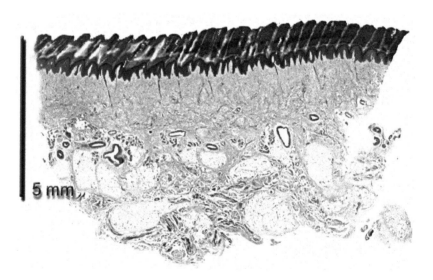

Figure 22
Skin biopsy from acromegalic patient showing marked epidermal hyperplasia,
a compacted dermis, thickened hypodermal connective tissue, and a
hyperplastic deep vascular plexus between the dermis and hypodermis.
Source: A. Beckers and G. Piérard

the key cardiovascular, respiratory, metabolic, musculoskeletal, and psychological morbidities (58).

Cardiovascular Complications

Acromegaly is associated with cardiomyopathy and related functional deficits and high rates of valvular disease, arrhythmias, and hypertension (58). The nature of acromegalic cardiomyopathy has been the subject of debate for many years, and current opinion favors the concept that GH/IGF-I hypersecretion causes a specific acromegalic cardiomyopathy. This is characterized by concentric ventricular hypertrophy due to an increase in cardiac myocyte size. It has been suggested that the hypertrophy is preceded by a period of left ventricular hyperkinesis and increased cardiac output (59). Chronic exposure to elevated levels of GH/IGF-I is associated with interstitial fibrosis of myocytes, which may occur as a result of myocarditis and increased apoptosis (60). Young patients less than 30 years old are now increasingly viewed as being at risk of early left ventricular hypertrophy, which was present in one-fifth of patients in this age group. The rates of ventricular hypertrophy seen on cardiac echography rise with an increasing duration of the disease, being reported in over one-half of patients under 40 years of age and nearly three-fourths of those aged up to 60 years (61). The immediate functional correlates of ventricular hypertrophy in acromegaly are diastolic dysfunction (impaired filling), and impairment of exercise tolerance due to decreased ejection fraction (62–64). With continued activity of acromegaly, the profile of cardiac disease gradually moves to one of congestive cardiac failure, which can become severe and require transplantation (Figs. 23 and 24) (65). Reduction of GH/IGF-I levels is associated with a reversal of features of acromegalic cardiomyopathy in young patients, while it appears that in those with established cardiac disease, aspects of pathology are not modifiable by therapy (66).

Given the structural cardiac changes that occur in chronic acromegaly, it is not surprising that both valvular and conduction system abnormalities are prominent. Pereira et al. reported that in 40 acromegalic patients, valvular disease was more than three times more prevalent than in controls matched for demographics and cardiac function. About one-third of acromegalic patients had significant aortic regurgitation (versus 7% of controls), while significant mitral regurgitation occurred in 5% of patients (67). A larger study in Naples indicated that valvular disease is even more frequent, and is related to left ventricular hypertrophy (68). Even cured patients exhibited persistent valvular dysfunction, reinforcing the concept that long-term acromegalic heart disease is characterized by permanent structural and functional changes. Conduction defects are prevalent and are seen in up to 40% of patients (69). Ventricular arrhythmias are particularly prominent, and ventricular premature complexes increase with disease duration (70). Ventricular late potentials—a marker of

(A)   (B)

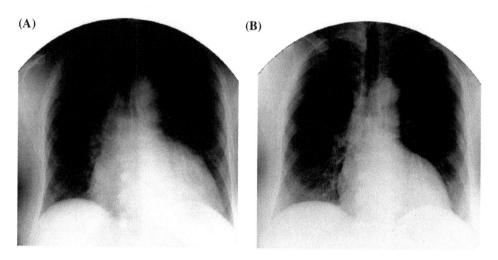

Figure 23
Chest radiograph in a 59-year-old female with acromegaly showing cardiome-
galy (**A**) that regressed following control of GH and IGF-I secretion (**B**).
Source: A. Beckers and P. Petrossians

clinically significant arrhythmias—are present in over one-half of acromegalic patients with uncontrolled disease (71).

Hypertension complicates up to 60% of cases of acromegaly (58), and
it has been recognized as a predictor of mortality in some series (1). As in
the general population, hypertension in acromegaly is usually multifactor-
ial in nature, with altered water and salt balance, vascular effects, and
metabolic elements all contributing to its presence and severity (72–75).

Respiratory Complications

The airway in acromegaly undergoes a series of changes due to the effects
of GH/IGF-I (76). Chest wall expansion leads to alterations in pulmonary
function, such as increased lung volumes, and compliance is also
increased, that together alter gas transfer (77,78). These alterations are
compounded by respiratory muscle myopathy, which forces the patient
to alter the pattern of breathing (79).

Upper airway changes to the larynx, pharynx, tongue, and mandible
leave the acromegalic patient at risk of airway occlusion, which may lead
to obstructive sleep apnea syndrome (80,81). These progressive deformities to the face and upper airway are shown in Figure 25. Persistent
obstructive sleep apnea is associated with decreased arterial oxygenation,
which in turn may predispose to hypertension and increased cardiovascular risk, which are both already enhanced (76). Obstructive sleep apnea is
amenable to therapy that improves airway architecture by decreasing soft
tissue swelling (76,82–85).

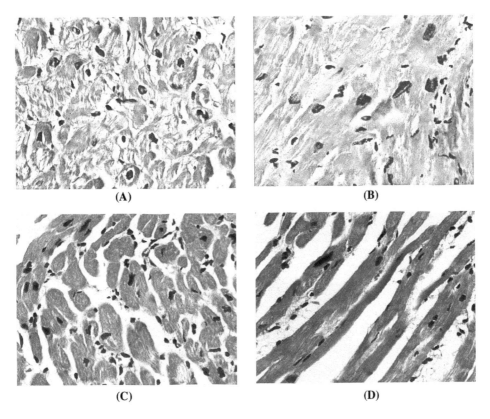

Figure 24
Cardiac muscle biopsies in an acromegalic patient with active disease showing
extensive myofibrillolysis, myocytosis, and infiltration (**A,B**). After control of
GH/IGF-I hypersecretion, a second cardiac biopsy shows extensive
improvement in pathological changes (**C,D**).
Source: A. Beckers and V. Legrand

Diabetes Mellitus

The antagonistic effects of GH on insulin action appear to overwhelm the
insulin-sensitizing effects of IGF-I in patients with acromegaly, leading
one-quarter to one-half of all patients to develop impaired glucose tolerance or frank diabetes mellitus (6,58,73). Acromegaly is associated with
insulin resistance, which occurs via a down-regulation by GH of the sensitivity of insulin receptors (via impairment of the function of the insulin
receptor substrate, IRS-1) (86). Thus, patients with acromegaly exhibit
impaired peripheral glucose uptake by skeletal muscle (87–90). These
effects produce alterations in the regulation of hepatic gluconeogenesis,
compounded by increased free fatty acid concentrations. Control of GH
secretion improves insulin sensitivity and decreases glucose resistance
and hyperinsulinemia (91).

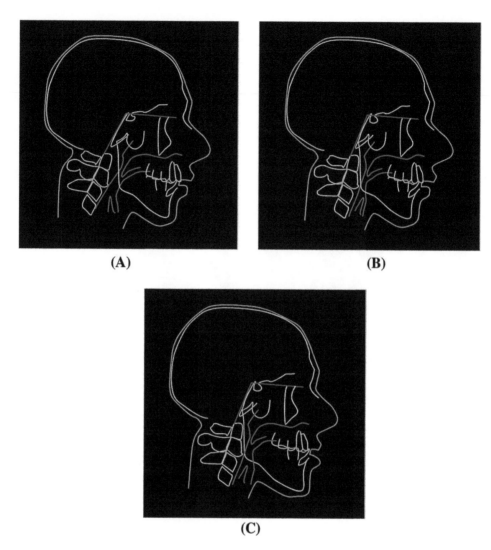

(A)   (B)

(C)

Figure 25
Upper airway architecture. (A) Normal upper airway with a craniobasal angle
(blue) of 118 degrees. (B) In acromegalic patients with a smaller craniobasal
angle, soft tissue swelling narrows the upper airway and increases the likelihood
of obstructive sleep apnea syndrome. (C) Prognathism further alters the upper
airway architecture.
Source: A. Beckers and P. Petrossians

Cancer

The incidence of cancer in patients with acromegaly has been one of the
most fiercely debated topics of the last decade. The growth-promoting
and anti-apoptotic effects of GH and IGF-I have been used to argue that
acromegaly represents a relatively permissive environment in which

neoplasia is more likely. Indeed, epidemiologic mortality studies have suggested an increased risk of cancer death in acromegalic patients (1). In a recent review of these data, Colao et al. (73) compared the prevalence of and mortality rates from cancer in acromegalic patients with the rates in the general U.S. population. They reported a total cancer prevalence of 10.9% (73), of which colorectal and thyroid cancers were notably higher compared with the general population. The overall mortality rate from cancer was 16.3% in acromegaly, with significantly higher individual rates for colorectal, thyroid, breast, soft tissue, and skin cancers when compared with the general population.

Much of the debate regarding cancer in acromegaly has centered on colorectal cancers, and acromegalic patients are thought to have double the risk of non-acromegalics for this cancer (92). Even in the largest and most conservative studies of cancer risk in acromegaly that do not support an *overall* increased rate, deaths from colorectal cancer outnumbered those in the general population quite clearly (93). Patients with acromegaly have increased rates of colonic polyps, which are considered to be at risk of undergoing malignant change (94). The data are conflicting on whether acromegalic patients in general have an increased risk of colonic polyps and colorectal cancer (92). Indeed, it appears that age plays a major role in determining colorectal polyp/cancer risk in acromegaly and that the risk is appreciably elevated only in male patients over 50 years of age. It appears that elevated GH and IGF-I levels are predictive of colorectal cancer risk, but the data are still not conclusive (73,95,96).

The most recent pragmatic suggestions for colorectal cancer screening in acromegalic patients without relevant signs/symptoms are a full colonoscopy at age 50, with follow-up every 3 years in cases where of colonic polyps are identified and removed, or every 5 years in cases with a clear initial colonoscopy (73).

Rheumatological Complications

Articular cartilages are a target for both GH and IGF-I. The combined effects of both can induce chondrocyte activity, which may eventually lead to thickening; these effects can be reversed somewhat by GH/IGF-I control (97,98). Joint distortion occurs as a result of the effects of GH/IGF-I in increasing cartilaginous thickness, enhancing joint laxity due to collagen mobilization, and promoting synovial overgrowth. Joint instability and abnormal load distribution on articular surfaces can lead to damage and increased calcification during repair (73). Bone also undergoes pathological changes in acromegaly, with the formation of osteophytes, particularly in the vertebrae. Disease pathology involves virtually all joints, leading to decreased mobility, pain, and physical deformity (e.g., kyphosis).

Quality of Life

Chronic illnesses have a negative impact on mood and psychological performance measures. This occurs because of a combination of factors that enhance the burden of disease, such as pain; disfigurement; limitation of social, work, and home life; isolation; and the necessity for treatment. In recent times, more interest has been paid to measuring these indicators in addition to harder biochemical or pathological endpoints in acromegaly. Quality of life (QOL) is a general term used to describe a patient's subjective rating of how a disease impacts or does not impact his or her life, responsibilities, and interests. Specific measures of QOL scores have been designed and validated in acromegaly. ACROQOL was developed from generic health-related QOL measures as a disease-specific QOL tool for use in acromegaly (99,100). Beyond the initial validation steps, few data have been published using ACROQOL. Recently Biermasz et al. (101) reported the use of QOL scales in patients with cured acromegaly (102). In 118 patients in remission, generic QOL measures showed significantly worse ratings for physical/social functioning, limitations due to physical/emotional problems, general health perception, fatigue, energy, pain, physical ability, anxiety, and depression compared with a control population standard. Radiotherapy was associated with lower QOL scores among cured patients, mainly in terms of greater fatigue, whereas somatostatin analog treatment was not associated with improved QOL scoring. Using a linear regression analysis, age predicted poorer physical subscales, and disease duration predicted social isolation and poorer social relations, while radiotherapy predicted poorer physical subscale performance and fatigue. These results have a high impact given that the patients had inactive disease and even worse scores would be expected in those with active disease. This indicates that improvement or normalization of QOL scores in acromegaly may represent a new goal for treatment. A further report from the same group indicates that important determinants of decreased QOL in cured patients include joint disease and myocardial infarction (102). One important factor to bear in mind is that established cardiovascular disease and arthropathy in acromegaly induce permanent changes that are relatively resistant to treatment (73).

REFERENCES

1. Holdaway IM, Rajasoorya C. Epidemiology of acromegaly. Pituitary 1999; 2(1):29–41.
2. Etxabe J, Gaztambide S, Latorre P, Vazquez JA. Acromegaly: an epidemiological study. J Endocrinol Invest 1993; 16(3):181–187.

3. Ritchie CM, Atkinson AB, Kennedy AL, Lyons AR, Gordon DS, Fannin T, Hadden DR. Ascertainment and natural history of treated acromegaly in Northern Ireland. Ulster Med J 1990; 59(1):55–62.

4. Bengtsson BA, Eden S, Ernest I, Oden A, Sjogren B. Epidemiology and long-term survival in acromegaly. A study of 166 cases diagnosed between 1955 and 1984. Acta Med Scand 1988; 223(4):327–335.

5. Alexander L, Appleton D, Hall R, Ross WM, Wilkinson R. Epidemiology of acromegaly in the Newcastle region. Clin Endocrinol (Oxf) 1980; 12(1): 71–79.

6. Mestron A, Webb SM, Astorga R, Benito P, Catala M, Gaztambide S, Gomez JM, Halperin I, Lucas-Morante T, Moreno B, Obiols G, de Pablos P, Paramo C, Pico A, Torres E, Varela C, Vazquez JA, Zamora J, Albareda M, Gilabert M. Epidemiology, clinical characteristics, outcome, morbidity and mortality in acromegaly based on the Spanish Acromegaly Registry (Registro Español de Acromegalia, REA). Eur J Endocrinol 2004; 151(4): 439–446.

7. Nabarro JD. Acromegaly. Clin Endocrinol (Oxf) 1987; 26(4):481–512.

8. Bates AS, Van't Hoff W, Jones JM, Clayton RN. An audit of outcome of treatment in acromegaly. Q J Med 1993; 86(5):293–299.

9. Rajasoorya C, Holdaway IM, Wrightson P, Scott DJ, Ibbertson HK. Determinants of clinical outcome and survival in acromegaly. Clin Endocrinol (Oxf) 1994; 41(1):95–102.

10. Wright AD, Hill DM, Lowy C, Fraser TR. Mortality in acromegaly. Q J Med 1970; 39(153):1–16.

11. Swearingen B, Barker FG, Katznelson L, Biller BM, Grinspoon S, Klibanski A, Moayeri N, Black PM, Zervas NT. Long-term mortality after transsphenoidal surgery and adjunctive therapy for acromegaly. J Clin Endocrinol Metab 1998; 83(10):3419–3426.

12. Beauregard C, Truong U, Hardy J, Serri O. Long-term outcome and mortality after transsphenoidal adenomectomy for acromegaly. Clin Endocrinol (Oxf) 2003; 58(1):86–91.

13. Arita K, Kurisu K, Tominaga A, Eguchi K, Iida K, Uozumi T, Kasagi F. Mortality in 154 surgically treated patients with acromegaly—a 10-year follow-up survey. Endocr J 2003; 50(2):163–172.

14. Ayuk J, Clayton RN, Holder G, Sheppard MC, Stewart PM, Bates AS. Growth hormone and pituitary radiotherapy, but not serum insulin-like growth factor-I concentrations, predict excess mortality in patients with acromegaly. J Clin Endocrinol Metab 2004; 89(4):1613–1617.

15. Holdaway IM, Rajasoorya RC, Gamble GD. Factors influencing mortality in acromegaly. J Clin Endocrinol Metab 2004; 89(2):667–674.

16. Biermasz NR, Dekker FW, Pereira AM, van Thiel SW, Schutte PJ, van Dulken H, Romijn JA, Roelfsema F. Determinants of survival in treated acromegaly in a single center: predictive value of serial insulin-like growth factor I measurements. J Clin Endocrinol Metab 2004; 89(6):2789–2796.

17. Asa SL, Kovacs K. Pituitary pathology in acromegaly. Endocrinol Metab Clin North Am 1992; 21(3):553–574.

18. Kovacs K, Horvath E, Vidal S. Classification of pituitary adenomas. J Neurooncol 2001; 54(2):121–127.

19. Horvath E, Kovacs K. Ultrastructural diagnosis of human pituitary adenomas. Microsc Res Tech 1992; 20(2):107–135.

20. Asa SL, Ezzat S. The cytogenesis and pathogenesis of pituitary adenomas. Endocr Rev 1998; 19(6):798–827.

21. Yamada S, Aiba T, Sano T, Kovacs K, Shishiba Y, Sawano S, Takada K. Growth hormone-producing pituitary adenomas: correlations between clinical characteristics and morphology. Neurosurgery 1993; 33(1):20–27.

22. Bando H, Sano T, Ohshima T, Zhang CY, Yamasaki R, Matsumoto K, Saito S. Differences in pathological findings and growth hormone responses in patients with growth hormone-producing pituitary adenoma. Endocrinol Jpn 1992; 39(4):355–363.

23. Ragel BT, Couldwell WT. Pituitary carcinoma: a review of the literature. Neurosurg Focus 2004; 16(4):E7.

24. Asa SL, Ezzat S. The pathogenesis of pituitary tumours. Nat Rev Cancer 2002; 2(11):836–849.

25. Barlier A, Gunz G, Zamora AJ, Morange-Ramos I, Figarella-Branger D, Dufour H, Enjalbert A, Jaquet P. Pronostic and therapeutic consequences of Gs alpha mutations in somatotroph adenomas. J Clin Endocrinol Metab 1998; 83(5):1604–1610.

26. Qian ZR, Sano T, Asa SL, Yamada S, Horiguchi H, Tashiro T, Li CC, Hirokawa M, Kovacs K, Ezzat S. Cytoplasmic expression of fibroblast growth factor receptor-4 in human pituitary adenomas: relation to tumor type, size, proliferation, and invasiveness. J Clin Endocrinol Metab 2004; 89(4):1904–1911.

27. Ezzat S, Zheng L, Asa SL. Pituitary tumor-derived fibroblast growth factor receptor 4 isoform disrupts neural cell-adhesion molecule/N-cadherin signaling to diminish cell adhesiveness: a mechanism underlying pituitary neoplasia. Mol Endocrinol 2004; 18(10):2543–2552.

28. Yu S, Asa SL, Weigel RJ, Ezzat S. Pituitary tumor AP-2alpha recognizes a cryptic promoter in intron 4 of fibroblast growth factor receptor 4. J Biol Chem 2003; 278(22):19597–19602.

29. Ezzat S, Zheng L, Zhu XF, Wu GE, Asa SL. Targeted expression of a human pituitary tumor-derived isoform of FGF receptor-4 recapitulates pituitary tumorigenesis. J Clin Invest 2002; 109(1):69–78.

30. Hunter JA, Skelly RH, Aylwin SJ, Geddes JF, Evanson J, Besser GM, Monson JP, Burrin JM. The relationship between pituitary tumour transforming gene (PTTG) expression and in vitro hormone and vascular endothelial growth factor (VEGF) secretion from human pituitary adenomas. Eur J Endocrinol 2003; 148(2):203–211.

31. McCabe CJ, Khaira JS, Boelaert K, Heaney AP, Tannahill LA, Hussain S, Mitchell R, Olliff J, Sheppard MC, Franklyn JA, Gittoes NJ. Expression of

pituitary tumour transforming gene (PTTG) and fibroblast growth factor-2 (FGF-2) in human pituitary adenomas: relationships to clinical tumour behaviour. Clin Endocrinol (Oxf) 2003; 58(2):141–150.

32. Thakker RV, Pook MA, Wooding C, Boscaro M, Scanarini M, Clayton RN. Association of somatotrophinomas with loss of alleles on chromosome 11 and with gsp mutations. J Clin Invest 1993; 91(6):2815–2821.

33. Poncin J, Stevenaert A, Beckers A. Somatic MEN1 gene mutation does not contribute significantly to sporadic pituitary tumorigenesis. Eur J Endocrinol 1999; 140(6):573–576.

34. Beckers A, Betea D, Socin HV, Stevenaert A. The treatment of sporadic versus MEN1-related pituitary adenomas. J Intern Med 2003; 253(6): 599–605.

35. Agarwal SK, Lee BA, Sukhodolets KE, Kennedy PA, Obungu VH, Hickman AB, Mullendore ME, Whitten I, Skarulis MC, Simonds WF, Mateo C, Crabtree JS, Scacheri PC, Ji Y, Novotny EA, Garrett-Beal L, Ward JM, Libutti SK, Richard AH, Cerrato A, Parisi MJ, Santa A, Oliver B, Chandrasekharappa SC, Collins FS, Spiegel AM, Marx SJ. Molecular pathology of the MEN1 gene. Ann N Y Acad Sci 2004; 1014:189–198.

36. Verges B, Boureille F, Goudet P, Murat A, Beckers A, Sassolas G, Cougard P, Chambe B, Montvernay C, Calender A. Pituitary disease in MEN type 1 (MEN1): data from the France-Belgium MEN1 multicenter study. J Clin Endocrinol Metab 2002; 87(2):457–465.

37. Carney JA, Gordon H, Carpenter PC, Shenoy BV, Go VL. The complex of myxomas, spotty pigmentation, and endocrine overactivity. Medicine (Baltimore) 1985; 64(4):270–283.

38. Stratakis CA, Matyakhina L, Courkoutsakis N, Patronas N, Voutetakis A, Stergiopoulos S, Bossis I, Carney JA. Pathology and molecular genetics of the pituitary gland in patients with the 'complex of spotty skin pigmentation, myxomas, endocrine overactivity and schwannomas' (Carney complex). Front Horm Res 2004; 32:253–264.

39. Sandrini F, Kirschner LS, Bei T, Farmakidis C, Yasufuku-Takano J, Takano K, Prezant TR, Marx SJ, Farrell WE, Clayton RN, Groussin L, Bertherat J, Stratakis CA. PRKAR1A, one of the Carney complex genes, and its locus (17q22–24) are rarely altered in pituitary tumours outside the Carney complex. J Med Genet 2002; 39(12):e78.

40. Akintoye SO, Chebli C, Booher S, Feuillan P, Kushner H, Leroith D, Cherman N, Bianco P, Wientroub S, Robey PG, Collins MT. Characterization of gsp-mediated growth hormone excess in the context of McCune-Albright syndrome. J Clin Endocrinol Metab 2002; 87(11):5104–5112.

41. Soares BS, Frohman LA. Isolated familial somatotropinoma. Pituitary 2004; 7(2):95–101.

42. Luccio-Camelo DC, Une KN, Ferreira RE, Khoo SK, Nickolov R, Bronstein MD, Vaisman M, Teh BT, Frohman LA, Mendonca BB, Gadelha MR. A meiotic recombination in a new isolated familial somatotropinoma kindred. Eur J Endocrinol 2004; 150(5):643–648.

43. Gadelha MR, Une KN, Rohde K, Vaisman M, Kineman RD, Frohman LA. Isolated familial somatotropinomas: establishment of linkage to chromosome 11q13.1–11q13.3 and evidence for a potential second locus at chromosome 2p16–12. J Clin Endocrinol Metab 2000; 85(2):707–714.

44. Verloes A, Stevenaert A, Teh BT, Petrossians P, Beckers A. Familial acromegaly: case report and review of the literature. Pituitary 1999; 1(3–4):273–277.

45. Athanassiadi K, Exarchos D, Tsagarakis S, Bellenis I. Acromegaly caused by ectopic growth hormone-releasing hormone secretion by a carcinoid bronchial tumor: a rare entity. J Thorac Cardiovasc Surg 2004; 128(4): 631–632.

46. Boix E, Pico A, Pinedo R, Aranda I, Kovacs K. Ectopic growth hormone-releasing hormone secretion by thymic carcinoid tumour. Clin Endocrinol (Oxf) 2002; 57(1):131–134.

47. Jansson JO, Svensson J, Bengtsson BA, Frohman LA, Ahlman H, Wangberg B, Nilsson O, Nilsson M. Acromegaly and Cushing's syndrome due to ectopic production of GHRH and ACTH by a thymic carcinoid tumour: in vitro responses to GHRH and GHRP-6. Clin Endocrinol (Oxf) 1998; 48(2): 243–250.

48. Ezzat S, Ezrin C, Yamashita S, Melmed S. Recurrent acromegaly resulting from ectopic growth hormone gene expression by a metastatic pancreatic tumor. Cancer 1993; 71(1):66–70.

49. Melmed S, Ziel FH, Braunstein GD, Downs T, Frohman LA. Medical management of acromegaly due to ectopic production of growth hormone-releasing hormone by a carcinoid tumor. J Clin Endocrinol Metab 1988; 67(2):395–399.

50. Mitsuya K, Nakasu Y, Nioka H, Nakasu S. Ectopic growth hormone-releasing adenoma in the cavernous sinus—case report. Neurol Med Chir (Tokyo) 2004; 44(7):380–385.

51. Matsuno A, Katayama H, Okazaki R, Toriumi M, Tanaka H, Akashi M, Tanaka K, Murakami M, Tanaka H, Nagashima T. Ectopic pituitary adenoma in the sphenoid sinus causing acromegaly associated with empty sella. ANZ J Surg 2001; 71(8):495–498.

52. Gondim JA, Schops M, Ferreira E, Bulcao T, Mota JI, Silveira C. Acromegaly due to an ectopic pituitary adenoma in the sphenoid sinus. Acta Radiol 2004; 45(6):689–691.

53. Asa SL, Scheithauer BW, Bilbao JM, Horvath E, Ryan N, Kovacs K, Randall RV, Laws ER Jr, Singer W, Linfoot JA. A case for hypothalamic acromegaly: a clinicopathological study of six patients with hypothalamic gangliocytomas producing growth hormone-releasing factor. J Clin Endocrinol Metab 1984; 58(5):796–803.

54. Karges B, Pfaffle R, Boehm BO, Karges W. Acromegaly induced by growth hormone replacement therapy. Horm Res 2004; 61(4):165–169.

55. Smith DA, Perry PJ. The efficacy of ergogenic agents in athletic competition. Part II: Other performance-enhancing agents. Ann Pharmacother 1992; 26(5):653–659.

56. Macintyre JG. Growth hormone and athletes. Sports Med 1987; 4(2): 129–142.

57. Minuto F, Barreca A, Melioli G. Indirect evidence of hormone abuse. Proof of doping? J Endocrinol Invest 2003; 26(9):919–923.

58. Giustina A, Casanueva FF, Cavagnini F, Chanson P, Clemmons D, Frohman LA, Gaillard R, Ho K, Jaquet P, Kleinberg DL, Lamberts SW, Lombardi G, Sheppard M, Strasburger CJ, Vance ML, Wass JA, Melmed S. Diagnosis and treatment of acromegaly complications. J Endocrinol Invest 2003; 26(12):1242–1247.

59. Vitale G, Pivonello R, Lombardi G, Colao A. Cardiovascular complications in acromegaly. Minerva Endocrinol 2004; 29(3):77–88.

60. Frustaci A, Chimenti C, Setoguchi M, Guerra S, Corsello S, Crea F, Leri A, Kajstura J, Anversa P, Maseri A. Cell death in acromegalic cardiomyopathy. Circulation 1999; 99(11):1426–1434.

61. Clayton RN. Cardiovascular function in acromegaly. Endocr Rev 2003; 24(3):272–277.

62. Ozbey N, Oncul A, Bugra Z, Vural A, Erzengin F, Orhan Y, Buyukozturk K, Sencer E, Molvalilar S. Acromegalic cardiomyopathy: evaluation of the left ventricular diastolic function in the subclinical stage. J Endocrinol Invest 1997; 20(6):305–311.

63. Cuocolo A, Nicolai E, Fazio S, Pace L, Maurea S, Cittadini A, Sacca L, Salvatore M. Impaired left ventricular diastolic filling in patients with acromegaly: assessment with radionuclide angiography. J Nucl Med 1995; 36(2):196–201.

64. Bertoni PD, Morandi G. Impaired left ventricular diastolic function in acromegaly: an echocardiographic study. Acta Cardiol 1987; 42(1):1–10.

65. Bihan H, Espinosa C, Valdes-Socin H, Salenave S, Young J, Levasseur S, Assayag P, Beckers A, Chanson P. Long-term outcome of patients with acromegaly and congestive heart failure. J Clin Endocrinol Metab 2004; 89(11):5308–5313.

66. Colao A, Marzullo P, Cuocolo A, Spinelli L, Pivonello R, Bonaduce D, Salvatore M, Lombardi G. Reversal of acromegalic cardiomyopathy in young but not in middle-aged patients after 12 months of treatment with the depot long-acting somatostatin analogue octreotide. Clin Endocrinol (Oxf) 2003; 58(2):169–176.

67. Pereira AM, van Thiel SW, Lindner JR, Roelfsema F, van der Wall EE, Morreau H, Smit JW, Romijn JA, Bax JJ. Increased prevalence of regurgitant valvular heart disease in acromegaly. J Clin Endocrinol Metab 2004; 89(1):71–75.

68. Colao A, Spinelli L, Marzullo P, Pivonello R, Petretta M, Di Somma C, Vitale G, Bonaduce D, Lombardi G. High prevalence of cardiac valve disease in acromegaly: an observational, analytical, case-control study. J Clin Endocrinol Metab 2003; 88(7):3196–3201.

69. Rodrigues EA, Caruana MP, Lahiri A, Nabarro JD, Jacobs HS, Raftery EB. Subclinical cardiac dysfunction in acromegaly: evidence for a specific disease of heart muscle. Br Heart J 1989; 62(3):185–194.

70. Kahaly G, Olshausen KV, Mohr-Kahaly S, Erbel R, Boor S, Beyer J, Meyer J. Arrhythmia profile in acromegaly. Eur Heart J 1992; 13(1):51–56.

71. Herrmann BL, Bruch C, Saller B, Ferdin S, Dagres N, Ose C, Erbel R, Mann K. Occurrence of ventricular late potentials in patients with active acromegaly. Clin Endocrinol (Oxf) 2001; 55(2):201–207.

72. Rizzoni D, Porteri E, Giustina A, De Ciuceis C, Sleiman I, Boari GE, Castellano M, Muiesan ML, Bonadonna S, Burattin A, Cerudelli B, Agabiti-Rosei E. Acromegalic patients show the presence of hypertrophic remodeling of subcutaneous small resistance arteries. Hypertension 2004; 43(3):561–565.

73. Colao A, Ferone D, Marzullo P, Lombardi G. Systemic complications of acromegaly: epidemiology, pathogenesis, and management. Endocr Rev 2004; 25(1):102–152.

74. Kreze A, Kreze-Spirova E, Mikulecky M. Risk factors for glucose intolerance in active acromegaly. Braz J Med Biol Res 2001; 34(11):1429–1433.

75. Pietrobelli DJ, Akopian M, Olivieri AO, Renauld A, Garrido D, Artese R, Feldstein CA. Altered circadian blood pressure profile in patients with active acromegaly. Relationship with left ventricular mass and hormonal values. J Hum Hypertens 2001; 15(9):601–605.

76. Fatti LM, Scacchi M, Pincelli AI, Lavezzi E, Cavagnini F. Prevalence and pathogenesis of sleep apnea and lung disease in acromegaly. Pituitary 2001; 4(4):259–262.

77. Donnelly PM, Grunstein RR, Peat JK, Woolcock AJ, Bye PT. Large lungs and growth hormone: an increased alveolar number? Eur Respir J 1995; 8(6):938–947.

78. Evans CC, Hipkin LJ, Murray GM. Pulmonary function in acromegaly. Thorax 1977; 32(3):322–327.

79. Iandelli I, Gorini M, Duranti R, Bassi F, Misuri G, Pacini F, Rosi E, Scano G. Respiratory muscle function and control of breathing in patients with acromegaly. Eur Respir J 1997; 10(5):977–982.

80. Dostalova S, Sonka K, Smahel Z, Weiss V, Marek J, Horinek D. Craniofacial abnormalities and their relevance for sleep apnoea syndrome aetiopathogenesis in acromegaly. Eur J Endocrinol 2001; 144(5):491–497.

81. Hochban W, Ehlenz K, Conradt R, Brandenburg U. Obstructive sleep apnoea in acromegaly: the role of craniofacial changes. Eur Respir J 1999; 14(1):196–202.

82. Herrmann BL, Wessendorf TE, Ajaj W, Kahlke S, Teschler H, Mann K. Effects of octreotide on sleep apnoea and tongue volume (magnetic resonance imaging) in patients with acromegaly. Eur J Endocrinol 2004; 151(3):309–315.

83. Ip MS, Tan KC, Peh WC, Lam KS. Effect of Sandostatin LAR on sleep apnoea in acromegaly: correlation with computerized tomographic cephalometry and hormonal activity. Clin Endocrinol (Oxf) 2001; 55(4):477–483.

84. Saeki N, Isono S, Tanaka A, Nishino T, Higuchi Y, Uchino Y, Iuchi T, Murai H, Tatsuno I, Yasuda T, Yamaura A. Pre- and post-operative respiratory assessment of acromegalics with sleep apnea–bedside oximetric study for transsphenoidal approach. Endocr J 2000; 47 (suppl:S61–4):S61–S64.

85. Saeki N, Isono S, Nishino T, Iuchi T, Yamaura A. Sleep-disordered breathing in acromegalics—relation of hormonal levels and quantitative sleep study by means of bedside oximeter. Endocr J 1999; 46(4):585–590.

86. Clemmons DR. Roles of insulin-like growth factor-I and growth hormone in mediating insulin resistance in acromegaly. Pituitary 2002; 5(3):181–183.

87. Moller N, Schmitz O, Joorgensen JO, Astrup J, Bak JF, Christensen SE, Alberti KG, Weeke J. Basal- and insulin-stimulated substrate metabolism in patients with active acromegaly before and after adenomectomy. J Clin Endocrinol Metab 1992; 74(5):1012–1019.

88. Foss MC. Peripheral glucose metabolism in healthy subjects and in endocrine diseases. Braz J Med Biol Res 1994; 27(4):959–979.

89. Foss MC, Saad MJ, Moreira AC. Peripheral muscle glucose and potassium transport in acromegaly. Horm Metab Res 1993; 25(1):45–47.

90. Foss MC, Saad MJ, Paccola GM, Paula FJ, Piccinato CE, Moreira AC. Peripheral glucose metabolism in acromegaly. J Clin Endocrinol Metab 1991; 72(5):1048–1053.

91. Drake WM, Rowles SV, Roberts ME, Fode FK, Besser GM, Monson JP, Trainer PJ. Insulin sensitivity and glucose tolerance improve in patients with acromegaly converted from depot octreotide to pegvisomant. Eur J Endocrinol 2003; 149(6):521–527.

92. Renehan AG, O'Connell J, O'Halloran D, Shanahan F, Potten CS, O'dwyer ST, Shalet SM. Acromegaly and colorectal cancer: a comprehensive review of epidemiology, biological mechanisms, and clinical implications. Horm Metab Res 2003; 35(11–12):712–725.

93. Orme SM, McNally RJ, Cartwright RA, Belchetz PE. Mortality and cancer incidence in acromegaly: a retrospective cohort study. United Kingdom Acromegaly Study Group. J Clin Endocrinol Metab 1998; 83(8):2730–2734.

94. Delhougne B, Deneux C, Abs R, Chanson P, Fierens H, Laurent-Puig P, Duysburgh I, Stevenaert A, Tabarin A, Delwaide J, Schaison G, Belaiche J, Beckers A. The prevalence of colonic polyps in acromegaly: a colonoscopic and pathological study in 103 patients. J Clin Endocrinol Metab 1995; 80(11):3223–3226.

95. Renehan AG, Shalet SM. Acromegaly and colorectal cancer: risk assessment should be based on population-based studies. J Clin Endocrinol Metab 2002; 87(4):1909.

96. Jenkins PJ, Frajese V, Jones AM, Camacho-Hubner C, Lowe DG, Fairclough PD, Chew SL, Grossman AB, Monson JP, Besser GM. Insulin-like growth factor I and the development of colorectal neoplasia in acromegaly. J Clin Endocrinol Metab 2000; 85(9):3218–3221.

97. Lieberman SA, Bjorkengren AG, Hoffman AR. Rheumatologic and skeletal changes in acromegaly. Endocrinol Metab Clin North Am 1992; 21(3): 615–631.

98. Colao A, Marzullo P, Vallone G, Marino V, Annecchino M, Ferone D, De Brasi D, Scarpa R, Oriente P, Lombardi G. Reversibility of joint thickening in acromegalic patients: an ultrasonography study. J Clin Endocrinol Metab 1998; 83(6):2121–2125.

99. Badia X, Webb SM, Prieto L, Lara N. Acromegaly Quality of Life Questionnaire (AcroQoL). Health Qual Life Outcomes 2004; 2(1):13.

100. Webb SM, Prieto L, Badia X, Albareda M, Catala M, Gaztambide S, Lucas T, Paramo C, Pico A, Lucas A, Halperin I, Obiols G, Astorga R. Acromegaly Quality of Life Questionnaire (ACROQOL) a new health-related quality of life questionnaire for patients with acromegaly: development and psychometric properties. Clin Endocrinol (Oxf) 2002; 57(2):251–258.

101. Biermasz NR, van Thiel SW, Pereira AM, Hoftijzer HC, van Hemert AM, Smit JW, Romijn JA, Roelfsema F. Decreased quality of life in patients with acromegaly despite long-term cure of growth hormone excess. J Clin Endocrinol Metab 2004; 89(11):5369–5376.

102. Biermasz NR, Pereira AM, Smit JW, Romijn JA, Roelfsema F. Morbidity after long-term remission for acromegaly; persisting joint-related complaints cause reduced quality of life. J Clin Endocrinol Metab 2005; 90(5):2731–2739.

Section II

DIAGNOSIS

Clinical, Endocrine and Radiologic Diagnosis of Acromegaly

INTRODUCTION

Acromegaly, like all diseases of insidious onset, requires a high index of clinical suspicion if it is to be detected early. The challenge to the physician is the ability to tie together sometimes nonspecific signs and symptoms involving various organ systems at an early stage in the disease process. The association of increased mortality and elevated growth hormone (GH) and insulin-like growth factor-I (IGF-I) levels (1), together with the knowledge that hormonal control is accompanied by normalization of mortality rates, provides a major impetus to diagnose patients as early as possible. Diagnosis of acromegaly is composed of three elements: identification of clinical signs and symptoms, performance of endocrine testing according to modern consensus criteria, and neuroradiological grading of the pituitary tumor using magnetic resonance imaging (MRI).

CLINICAL DIAGNOSIS AND WORKUP

As described in previous chapters, chronic hypersecretion of GH and IGF-I leads to clinically significant changes in virtually all organ systems. The physical features of the patient with well-established acromegaly are

Table 1
Prevalence of Signs and Symptoms of Acromegaly in a Series of 500 Patients[a]

<30%	30–60%	>60%
Depression	Headache	Acral growth
Reduced libido	Erectile dysfunction	Deformity of facial
Carpal tunnel syndrome	Arthritis	features
Daytime somnolence	Asthenia/fatigue	Soft tissue swelling
Myopathy	Peripheral neuropathy	Increased sweating
Increased hair growth	Paresthesia	
Dyspnea/breathlessness		
Galactorrhea		

[a]Signs and symptoms were graded as mild, moderate, or severe.
Source: From Ref. 3.

virtually pathognomonic. In contrast, early acromegaly may be characterized by nonspecific complaints, such as increased sweating, mild soft tissue swelling, or decreased energy. The frequency of various signs and
symptoms in acromegaly has been reported in some larger case collec-
tions (Table 1) (2–4). From these data we can see that patients almost
invariably report acral growth and changes in facial features, although
important but nonspecific problems, such as decreased libido, impaired
erectile function, and fatigue are also very prominent (3). These studies,
while informative, describe the disease activity of acromegaly in patients
treated from 1963 until 1990. In many cases, these patients were diagnosed in an era before newer medical therapies, when the impact of hormonal control on mortality was unknown. It is to be hoped that earlier
diagnosis and tighter hormonal control of acromegaly will reduce the
disease burden suffered by patients before a diagnosis is made.

Acral Growth

Abnormal growth of the hands or feet in adulthood is a cardinal symptom
of acromegaly that is reported to some degree by the overwhelming
majority of patients in large historical series (2,3). Few, if any, other conditions are associated with the acral growth typical of acromegaly in
which patients report successive changes in shoe or ring size (Fig. 1).
Acral growth is predominantly caused by soft tissue swelling, which
increases the width of the fingers, hands, and feet; osteoarthritis and joint
hyperlaxity can also contribute to hand deformity (Fig. 2). Patients may
report that shoes become too narrow or must seek extra-wide fitting shoes
due to the abnormal shape of their feet (Fig. 3).

Face and Oral Cavity

The patient presenting with typical acromegalic facies does not represent
an enormous diagnostic challenge (Fig. 4). Late de novo presentation with

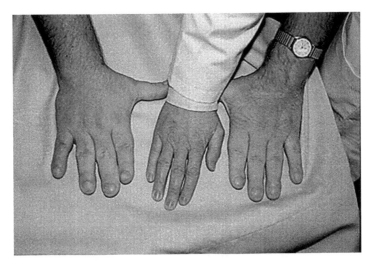

Figure 1
Typical enlargement of the hands in acromegaly. In comparison with a
normal hand (*center*), the hands of a patient with established acromegaly are
significantly broadened.
Source: A. Beckers

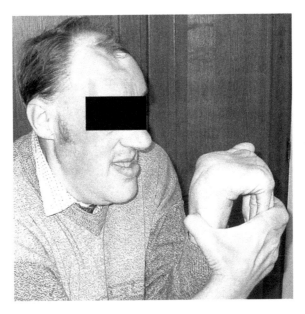

Figure 2
Joint hyperlaxity in acromegaly. Chronic overactivity of the GH–IGF-I axis
in acromegaly leads to articular changes, which can destabilize joints. In
the hand, hyperlaxity as part of arthropathy can contribute to the deformation
typically associated with established acromegaly.
Source: A. Beckers

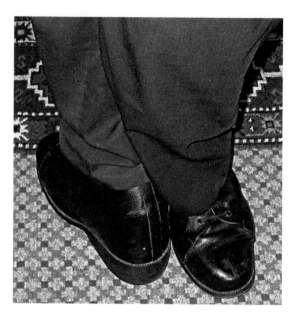

Figure 3
Effects of lower limb acral deformity. Chronic hypersecretion of GH/IGF-I in this patient has led to deformities of the feet, necessitating the wearing of specially adapted widened shoes. Hyperlaxity of the hip joint permits the patient to readily assume the abnormal foot posture shown in the image.
Source: A. Beckers

advanced disease should become increasingly rare in the future in the developed world. Typical components of the coarsened features seen in acromegaly, such as prognathism and prominence of the brow, may be subtler in younger patients. For example, the patient depicted in Figure 5A demonstrates furrowing of the forehead, enlargement of the nose, and generalized mild soft tissue swelling; the profile view is relatively unremarkable (Fig. 5B). Another young patient shown in Figure 6 has mild prognathism and soft tissue swelling of the face, although neither physical sign is very marked.

Macroglossia usually accompanies the facial changes seen in patients with established acromegaly (Fig. 7). Increased interdental spacing should raise strong suspicions of acromegaly (Fig. 8), and such a finding has led to referrals to endocrinologists by dental practitioners (2). In combination with macroglossia and prognathism (Fig. 9), swelling of the pharyngeal tissues can occur. These alterations in oropharyngeal architecture contribute greatly to upper airway obstruction in sleep apnea syndrome. Thus, the occurrence of excessive snoring and daytime somnolence should be queried to the patient and their family.

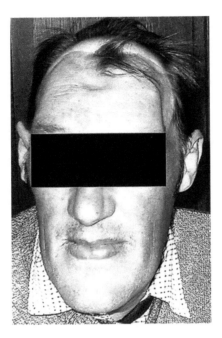

Figure 4

Acromegalic facies. Prognathism and frontal bossing are evident in this patient, who has long-term hypersecretion of GH and IGF-I.
Source: A. Beckers

Skin and Appendices

Profound skin changes are characteristic of acromegaly and contribute to facial and acral deformities. The skin undergoes pathological changes in terms of connective tissue and the extracellular matrix, which leads to altered tensile properties and thickening (5–8). In some cases the skin thickening can become extremely pronounced; this is termed *cutis verticis gyrata* and is characterized by deeply folded ridges on the scalp and forehead, which may be visible on a CT scan (9–11).

Increased sweating is characteristic of acromegaly and derives in part from significantly increased sweat gland size and richer sudomotor innervation (12,13). Sneppen et al. (14) have suggested that increased sweat gland secretion may persist despite adequate control of GH and IGF-I secretion. The increase in sweat gland size also accounts for the increased oiliness and greasiness of the skin (Fig. 7) in addition to a propensity for strong body odor (15).

Excess skin tag formation is also common in acromegaly, and one study has suggested a correlation between skin tags and colonic polyps (16). Because acromegaly is associated with insulin resistance, patients should be examined for the velvety pigmentation of *acanthosis nigricans*, which occurs particularly in the axillae (2,17).

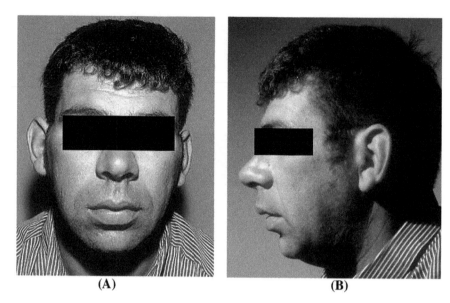

Figure 5
Facial features of a young patient with acromegaly. (**A**) The patient demonstrates relatively mild features of the disease with modest swelling of the lips, nose, and facial skin and furrowing of the forehead. (**B**) The profile view confirms the soft tissue swelling and the suggestion of an enlarged nose, but prognathism is noticeably absent.
Source: A. Beckers

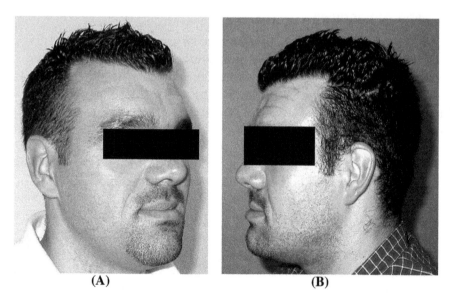

Figure 6
Moderate acromegalic facial features. (**A**) This young patient exhibits moderate soft tissue swelling around the mouth, cheeks, brow, and forehead. (**B**) The profile demonstrates prognathism, furrowing of the brow, and enhanced oiliness of the skin.
Source: A. Beckers

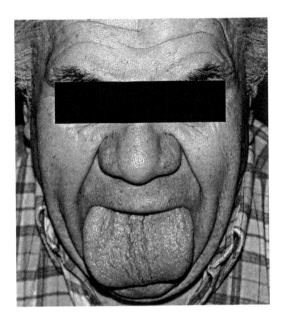

Figure 7
Macroglossia in acromegaly. This patient with established acromegaly
demonstrates macroglossia, soft tissue swelling, furrowing of the forehead,
and brow prominence. There is also evidence of increased
sebaceous secretion.
Source: A. Beckers

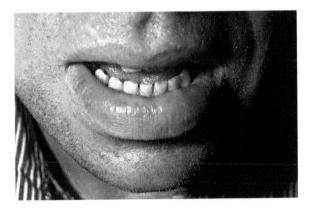

Figure 8
Increased interdental spacing in an acromegalic patient. This is one of the
cardinal signs of acromegaly and is mimicked by few other conditions.
Source: A. Beckers

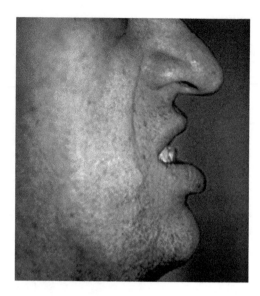

Figure 9
Prognathism in a patient with acromegaly.
Source: A. Beckers

Musculoskeletal System

Arthropathy is a common feature of acromegaly that occurs in up to 60% of patients (3). All joints can be affected, with more than 50% of patients suffering from spinal arthritis and reported limited movement in 56% of cases (18). About three-fourths of patients suffer from an abnormality of the appendicular skeleton (19). Patients with longer disease duration appear to have a greater arthritis burden, but joint abnormalities can also occur in younger patients (20). Patients with acromegaly commonly report that they have a low energy reserve and may fatigue easily (3). In the absence of demonstrable intercurrent cardiac or thyroid disease, this symptom may be due to proximal myopathy.

Respiratory System

Patients with acromegaly exhibit significant abnormalities of the respiratory system that may be evident on clinical examination and noninvasive functional testing (21). Probably the first noticeable pathology of the respiratory tract seen during the clinical examination is that of altered voice. Patients with acromegaly have a lower fundamental vocal frequency, which occurs as a result of increased vocal cord mass. This approaches normal after pituitary surgery and hormonal normalization (22). An increased anterior–posterior diameter of the thorax is evident in many patients with established disease (Fig. 10). This marked deformity of the chest wall overlies a series of respiratory tract abnormalities that can be measured readily in the hospital setting, and such information can be useful for the anesthetist (23,24). Pulmonary function testing may reveal increased lung volumes, particularly in vital capacity and total lung capacity; lung compliance is also increased (25). The carbon monoxide transfer coefficient (K_{CO}) may be decreased in patients with increased chest width and lung capacity (26), although some have found normal pulmonary diffusion capacity in the setting of enlarged lungs in acromegaly (27). Inspiratory and expiratory muscle function is abnormal in a significant proportion of acromegalic patients. Respiratory muscular force is decreased and patients may have a decreased inspiratory time, leading to increased frequency of respiration (28). Upper airway obstruction in acromegaly can occur in up to 50% of patients,

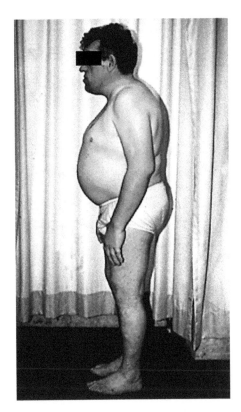

Figure 10
Increased anteroposterior diameter of the thorax. Patients with active acromegaly for many years can develop this major chest wall deformity, which leaves the patient with a "barrel chest." The consequences of this increased anteroposterior diameter are pathological alterations in lung volumes and respiratory muscle efficiency.
Source: A. Beckers

and the involved sites include the pharynx, hypopharynx, and larynx. Intrathoracic airway collapse is also reported (29). As previously noted, clinical assessment of the acromegalic patient should always include questioning of the patient and family about snoring and daytime somnolence as part of obstructive sleep apnea syndrome.

Cardiovascular System

The signs and symptoms of cardiovascular disease in acromegaly, while not specific, are of significant interest. Chronic GH/IGF-I excess leads to left ventricular hypertrophy and a series of alterations in cardiac structure (30). Left ventricular hypertrophy is an early finding in acromegaly (20) and should be actively sought and characterized during clinical workup using echocardiography. Such pathological changes, when they impair left ventricular filling and contraction, may be evident as the presence of a heave on examination of the precordium and as displacement of the cardiac apex. Left ventricular hypertrophy also leads to an increased risk of valvular lesions, particularly regurgitant aortic and mitral valves, which may persist despite hormonal control (31,32). Hypertension, defined as a diastolic pressure greater than 90 mmHg, has been reported to occur in 40% of patients–five times more frequently than in a corresponding control population (20). Arrhythmias, particularly those of ventricular origin, are more common in acromegaly than in the general population (33). Patients should be questioned about symptoms suggestive of significant cardiac rhythm disturbance (palpitations, syncope, etc.) and undergo an electrocardiogram during diagnostic workup. Acromegalic patient with chronically active disease and left ventricular abnormalities should have a 24-hr Holter monitor performed.

Nervous System

The most common neurological symptom of acromegaly is headache, which occurs in up to 60% of patients (3); headache severity is not necessarily proportionate to adenoma size. The local effects of a pituitary tumor on visual fields and acuity should be tested by confrontation and a Snellen chart, and fundoscopy should be performed. If a homonymous hemianopia or a quadrantanopia is suspected, follow-up with Goldmann perimetry should be pursued. The involvement of cranial nerves III, IV, V, and VI can occur in acromegaly when the cavernous sinus is invaded by a pituitary adenoma. The third cranial nerve is particularly vulnerable to lateral displacement by a large intrasellar tumor, leading to signs including ptosis, ophthalmoplegia, and abnormal pupillary reflexes.

Carpal tunnel syndrome is a classical peripheral neuropathy suffered by acromegalic patients and occurs to a moderate or severe degree in approximately 15% of cases (3). The syndrome was long thought to be due to soft tissue compression of the median nerve entering the hand at the level of the carpal bones. However, using serial MRI of the wrist and carpal tunnel contents, Jenkins et al. reported that median nerve edema was the predominant cause of the neuropathy in acromegaly, and the reduction in symptoms afforded by hormonal control was associated with a reduction in the edema (34). Evidence suggests that other peripheral nerves also undergo enlargement in active acromegaly, but these abnormalities are usually asymptomatic (35).

Endocrine and Metabolic Systems

Thyroid examination should be performed in all patients, as thyroid disorders are a frequent complication of acromegaly. One of the largest recent series suggests that a full 78% of acromegalic patients have concomitant thyroid disease, of which nearly 58% had a nontoxic goiter (36). Hyperthyroid states were present in about 15% of cases, and thyroid cancer occurred in 1.2% of patients (36).

During clinical examination, signs and symptoms of other pituitary pathologies should be sought for, particularly those related to hyperprolactinemia secondary to a GH/prolactin co-secreting pituitary adenoma. Hypopituitarism may occur secondary to invasion or expansion of a GH-secreting pituitary tumor, and effects on menstrual cycle, fertility, and libido may be useful indicators of hypogonadism, which occurs frequently in acromegaly (37).

Diabetes mellitus complicates acromegaly in 20–50% of cases, while a state of insulin resistance/glucose intolerance may be found in another 15–25% of cases; these reported rates vary depending on the criteria used to define disordered carbohydrate metabolism (2,3,38,39). The clinical examination of the acromegalic patient should include surveillance for secondary effects of uncontrolled diabetes mellitus, such as retinopathy, peripheral neuropathy, and poor wound healing in the lower limbs.

Cancer

Patients with acromegaly have an elevated risk of colorectal cancer from epidemiological studies (40,41), and evidence suggests that breast cancer survival may be decreased (20). Clinical assessment of the patient with acromegaly should incorporate relevant questioning and examination for signs or symptoms of these and other malignancies.

ENDOCRINE DIAGNOSIS

The endocrine diagnosis of acromegaly involves the performance of a series of appropriate static and dynamic biochemical tests of the GH–IGF-I axis. Proper interpretation of test results allows a diagnosis of acromegaly to be made or discounted relatively simply and in a timely manner. The biochemical diagnosis of acromegaly relies on an appreciation of the strengths and limitations of the assay systems used, particularly in terms of the lower limit of quantitation and the physiological/pathological factors that can skew assay results. These issues are of relevance for the measurement of GH and IGF-I in diagnosis.

Static Tests

For many years, basal GH levels were used in the biochemical diagnosis of acromegaly. Basal GH was taken as the lowest of a series of individual measures or as the lowest level during a timed series. Over time, the "acceptable" nadir level for GH decreased from $10\,\mu g/L$ to $5\,\mu g/L$ to $2\,\mu g/L$, until more sensitive assays demonstrated that acromegaly can exist in patients with nadir GH levels below 1 $\mu g/L$ (42–44). As such, a series of "normal" GH levels do not reliably exclude the presence of acromegaly. Other static tests including urinary GH, IGFBP-3, acid-labile subunit, and free IGF-I are not of proven value as diagnostic criteria. In the rare case where acromegaly is thought to be due to GHRH secretion by a peripheral endocrine-active tumor, GHRH levels should be measured.

Serum IGF-I Level

Significant improvements have been made over the years in the methodologies used to measure IGF-I, which have increased its reliability and usefulness in static diagnosis. IGF-I is an accurate reflection of the integrated effect of GH secretion (45) and is a reliable measure of disease activity in acromegaly (46). The availability of sizable datasets describing the IGF-I range for normal individuals stratified for age and sex is necessary for each assay system to determine whether an individual IGF-I result is above normal (47). Elevated serum IGF-I can be used to diagnose acromegaly in patients with minimal or borderline elevations of serum GH (48). Other static tests related to IGF-I, such as the measurement of IGFBP-3 or free IGF-I, are of limited value as they have not been shown to be superior to measuring total IGF-I.

During interpretation of test results, it should be kept in mind that IGF-I is increased during pregnancy and adolescence, and decreased by poorly controlled diabetes mellitus, malnutrition, liver disease, and severe renal failure (49). Ideally, each patient should be followed over time using the same validated IGF-I assay system to allow the clinician to judge the activity of acromegaly in response to various treatments.

Dynamic Tests

Many dynamic tests that rely on the stimulation or suppression of GH secretion have been used over the years. Of these, only the suppression of GH secretion during an oral glucose tolerance test (OGTT) remains in widespread use today. The thyrotropin releasing hormone (TRH) test and other hypothalamic hormone stimulatory tests do not provide significant added value over that provided by an OGTT and IGF-I level. However, these other stimulation tests as well as basal hormonal profiles are extremely valuable for the diagnosis of hypopituitarism associated with a GH-secreting pituitary adenoma.

Oral Glucose Tolerance Test (OGTT)

The failure to suppress GH to $<1\,\mu g/L$ during a 2 hr OGTT is the most frequent dynamic criterion used for the diagnosis of acromegaly (50). The patient fasts overnight, and the next morning an intravenous catheter is placed, preferably 30 min before the OGTT begins. The patient ingests 75 g of glucose at time 0 and blood samples for GH and glucose are taken at half-hourly intervals for 120 min. Interpretation of the OGTT in acromegaly can be skewed by the presence of diabetes mellitus, liver and renal disease, and anorexia nervosa, which can give false-positive results. Recent evidence has noted the existence of patients with active acromegaly despite "fully" suppressed GH levels (42–44); thus, post-OGTT GH results should ideally be paired with an age- and sex-matched IGF-I measurement.

RADIOLOGIC DIAGNOSIS

When the results of clinical examination and appropriate hormonal testing indicate the presence of acromegaly, radiological confirmation of a pituitary adenoma should be sought using MRI. Neuroradiological imaging is important not only to confirm the presence of a pituitary tumor, but also to classify its size, its site in the pituitary, its consistency (e.g., cystic), its relationship to surrounding structures, and whether extension/invasion has occurred. Enhancement with gadolinium is useful to help in the detection of microadenomas, and maximum enhancement of the pituitary adenoma on MRI occurs shortly (<5 min) after injection (51). GH-secreting pituitary macroadenomas have either low intensity or are isointense on T1-weighted series, while on T2-weighted images soft tumors have high signal intensity and solid tumors are more likely to be isointense (52).

MRI data are used for the classification of tumors by size into microadenomas (<10 mm in diameter) or macroadenomas (>10 mm in diameter), while giant pituitary adenomas have a maximum diameter of >40 mm. MRI examples of the normal pituitary region, microadenomas, macroadenomas, and a giant pituitary adenoma are shown in Figures 11–17.

A classification system for pituitary adenomas was developed using a combination of surgical findings and radiological images by Hardy, Vezina, and others (53), which has since been applied to MRI results. This scheme grades pituitary adenomas first according to the grades of associated sella turcica involvement. Grade 0 has a normal intact sella, which progresses through enclosed microadenomas (grade 1) and enclosed macroadenomas (grade 2) to invasive macroadenomas (grades 3 and 4), with increasing associated sella turcica abnormalities. This grading scheme is shown graphically in Figure 18. For tumors with extrasellar extension, a separate subclassification has been developed:

Suprasellar/symmetrical
  A. 10 mm: Fills the chiasmatic cistern
  B. 20 mm: Raises the third ventricle recesses
  C. >30 mm: Fills the anterior portion of the third ventricle

Parasellar/asymmetrical
  D. Extends intracranially
  E. Lateral extension outward from cavernous sinus

The importance of MRI data has been underlined by the finding that MRI characteristics of GH-secreting pituitary adenomas, such as tumor volume, extension, and invasion, are predictive of outcomes of transsphenoidal surgery in terms of disease control (54).

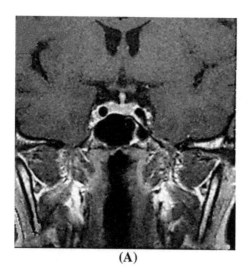
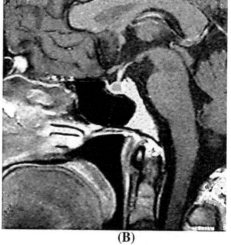

(A)   (B)

Figure 11

MRI of normal pituitary gland. (A) Coronal view. (B) Sagittal view.
Source: A. Beckers

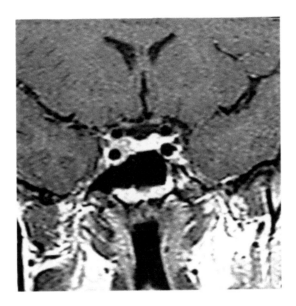

Figure 12
MRI of pituitary microadenoma. In this gadolinium contrast-enhanced image, a microadenoma is present on the right side of the pituitary.
Source: A. Beckers

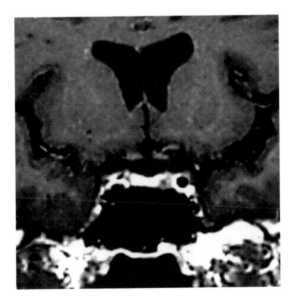

Figure 13
MRI of pituitary microadenoma. A left-sided microadenoma is shown in this contrast-enhanced image.
Source: A. Beckers

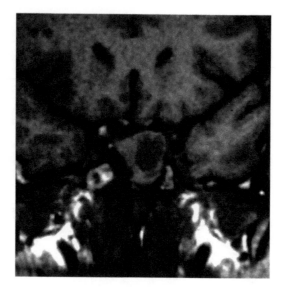

Figure 14
MRI of GH-secreting pituitary macroadenoma. The left upper portion of the
adenoma may be cystic, and some degree of chiasmal compression is present.
Source: A. Beckers and A. Stevenaert

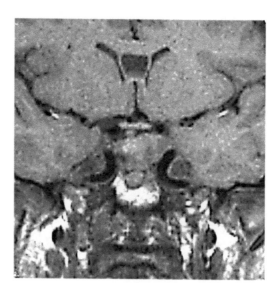

Figure 15
MRI of GH-secreting pituitary macroadenoma. In this case, the macroadenoma
does not impinge on the chiasma.
Source: A. Beckers and A. Stevenaert

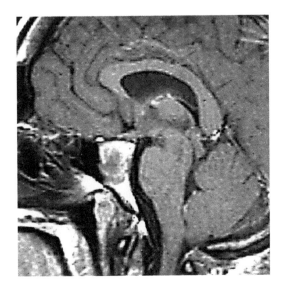

Figure 16
Sagittal MRI view of a GH-secreting pituitary macroadenoma.
Source: A. Beckers

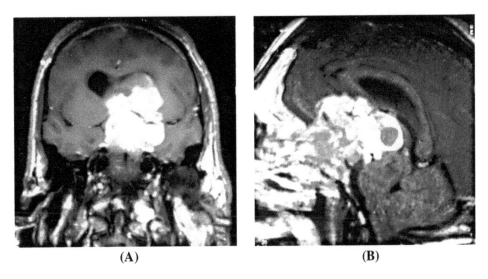

(A)   (B)

Figure 17
A giant GH-secreting pituitary adenoma. (**A**) This adenoma has extended
intracranially and obliterates the left lateral ventricle. (**B**) A sagittal view
demonstrates the heterogeneity of the consistency of the tumor on T1-weighted
imaging, with multiple cystic regions present.
Source: A. Beckers

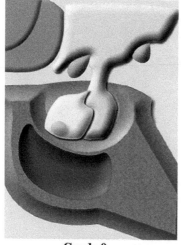

Grade 0

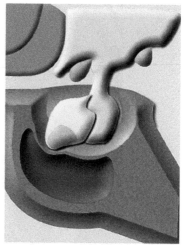

Grade 1

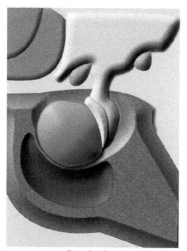

Grade 2

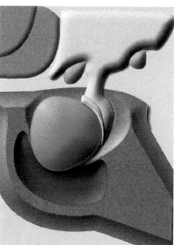

Grade 3

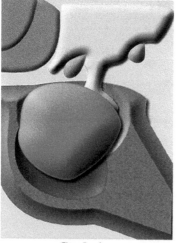

Grade 4

Figure 18
Schematic of the Hardy classification
of pituitary adenomas: *Grade 0*: Fully
contained intrasellar microadenoma.
Grade 1: Intrasellar microadenoma
with local sellar distortion. *Grade 2*:
Macroadenoma with global expansion
of the sella. *Grade 3*: macroadenoma
with local destruction of the floor of
the sella and invasion of the sphenoid
or cavernous sinuses. *Grade 4*: Macroadenoma with total sellar destruction
and local invasion.
Source: A. Beckers and P. Petrossians

Ectopic Tumors

For patients with acromegaly caused by ectopic GHRH (or *very* rarely GH) secretion due to a carcinoid, locating the primary tumor may require extensive radiological imaging of the head and neck, thorax, and abdomen (55–62). Ectopic GHRH secretion may also occur close to the pituitary, such as in the cavernous sinus (63). For occult lesions, somatostatin receptor scintigraphy may be useful (64), as many endocrine-active tumors express somatostatin receptors, particularly type 2, to which the radionuclide ^{111}In-DTPA-D-Phe(1) octreotide binds (65).

REFERENCES

1. Holdaway IM, Rajasoorya CR, Gamble GD, Stewart AW. Long-term treatment outcome in acromegaly. Growth Horm IGF Res 2003; 13(4):185–192.
2. Nabarro JD. Acromegaly. Clin Endocrinol (Oxf) 1987; 26(4):481–512.
3. Ezzat S, Forster MJ, Berchtold P, Redelmeier DA, Boerlin V, Harris AG. Acromegaly. Clinical and biochemical features in 500 patients. Medicine (Baltimore) 1994; 73(5):233–240.
4. Vance ML, Harris AG. Long-term treatment of 189 acromegalic patients with the somatostatin analog octreotide. Results of the International Multicenter Acromegaly Study Group. Arch Intern Med 1991; 151(8):1573–1578.
5. Matsuoka LY, Wortsman J, Kupchella CE, Eng A, Dietrich JE. Histochemical characterization of the cutaneous involvement of acromegaly. Arch Intern Med 1982; 142(10):1820–1823.
6. Quatresooz P, Hermanns-Le T, Ciccarelli A, Beckers A, Pierard GE. Tensegrity and type 1 dermal dendrocytes in acromegaly. Eur J Clin Invest 2005; 35(2):133–139.
7. Centurion SA, Schwartz RA. Cutaneous signs of acromegaly. Int J Dermatol 2002; 41(10):631–634.
8. Braham C, Betea D, Pierard-Franchimont C, Beckers A, Pierard GE. Skin tensile properties in patients treated for acromegaly. Dermatology 2002; 204(4):325–329.
9. Zangeneh F, Carpenter PC. Visual vignette. Cutis verticis gyrata (CVG) in acromegaly. Endocr Pract 2002; 8(6):475.
10. Kolawole TM, Al Orainy IA, Patel PJ, Fathuddin S. Cutis verticis gyrata: its computed tomographic demonstration in acromegaly. Eur J Radiol 1998; 27(2):145–148.
11. O'Reilly FM, Sliney I, O'Loughlin S. Acromegaly and cutis verticis gyrata. J R Soc Med 1997; 90(2):79.
12. Hasan W, Cowen T, Barnett PS, Elliot E, Coskeran P, Bouloux PM. The sweating apparatus in growth hormone deficiency, following treatment with r-hGH and in acromegaly. Auton Neurosci 2001; 2089(1–2):100–109.

13. Burton JL, Libman LJ, Cunliffe WJ, Wilkinson R, Hall R, Shuster S. Sebum excretion in acromegaly. Br Med J 1972; 1(797):406–408.

14. Sneppen SB, Main KM, Juul A, Pedersen LM, Kristensen LO, Skakkebaek NE, Feldt-Rasmussen U. Sweat secretion rates in growth hormone disorders. Clin Endocrinol (Oxf) 2000; 53(5):601–608.

15. Feingold KR, Elias PM. Endocrine–skin interactions. Cutaneous manifestations of pituitary disease, thyroid disease, calcium disorders, and diabetes. J Am Acad Dermatol 1987; 17(6):921–940.

16. Leavitt J, Klein I, Kendricks F, Gavaler J, Van Thiel DH. Skin tags: a cutaneous marker for colonic polyps. Ann Intern Med 1983; 98(6):928–930.

17. Brown J, Winkelmann RK, Randall RV. Acanthosis nigricans and pituitary tumors. Report of eight cases. JAMA 1966; 198(6):619–623.

18. Scarpa R, De Brasi D, Pivonello R, Marzullo P, Manguso F, Sodano A, Oriente P, Lombardi G, Colao A. Acromegalic axial arthropathy: a clinical case-control study. J Clin Endocrinol Metab 2004; 89(2):598–603.

19. Podgorski M, Robinson B, Weissberger A, Stiel J, Wang S, Brooks PM. Articular manifestations of acromegaly. Aust N Z J Med 1988; 18(1):28–35.

20. Colao A, Ferone D, Marzullo P, Lombardi G. Systemic complications of acromegaly: epidemiology, pathogenesis, and management. Endocr Rev 2004; 25(1):102–152.

21. Fatti LM, Scacchi M, Pincelli AI, Lavezzi E, Cavagnini F. Prevalence and pathogenesis of sleep apnea and lung disease in acromegaly. Pituitary 2001; 4(4):259–262.

22. Williams RG, Richards SH, Mills RG, Eccles R. Voice changes in acromegaly. Laryngoscope 1994; 104(4):484–487.

23. Smith M, Hirsch NP. Pituitary disease and anaesthesia. Br J Anaesth 2000; 85(1):3–14.

24. Hakala P, Randell T, Valli H. Laryngoscopy and fibreoptic intubation in acromegalic patients. Br J Anaesth 1998; 80(3):345–347.

25. Evans CC, Hipkin LJ, Murray GM. Pulmonary function in acromegaly. Thorax 1977; 32(3):322–327.

26. Donnelly PM, Grunstein RR, Peat JK, Woolcock AJ, Bye PT. Large lungs and growth hormone: an increased alveolar number? Eur Respir J 1995; 8(6):938–947.

27. Garcia-Rio F, Pino JM, Diez JJ, Ruiz A, Villasante C, Villamor J. Reduction of lung distensibility in acromegaly after suppression of growth hormone hypersecretion. Am J Respir Crit Care Med 2001; 164(5):852–857.

28. Iandelli I, Gorini M, Duranti R, Bassi F, Misuri G, Pacini F, Rosi E, Scano G. Respiratory muscle function and control of breathing in patients with acromegaly. Eur Respir J 1997; 10(5):977–982.

29. Trotman-Dickenson B, Weetman AP, Hughes JM. Upper airflow obstruction and pulmonary function in acromegaly: relationship to disease activity. Q J Med 1991; 79(290):527–538.

30. Clayton RN. Cardiovascular function in acromegaly. Endocr Rev 2003; 24(3):272–277.

31. Pereira AM, van Thiel SW, Lindner JR, Roelfsema F, van der Wall EE, Morreau H, Smit JW, Romijn JA, Bax JJ. Increased prevalence of regurgitant valvular heart disease in acromegaly. J Clin Endocrinol Metab 2004; 89(1): 71–75.

32. Colao A, Spinelli L, Marzullo P, Pivonello R, Petretta M, Di Somma C, Vitale G, Bonaduce D, Lombardi G. High prevalence of cardiac valve disease in acromegaly: an observational, analytical, case-control study. J Clin Endocrinol Metab 2003; 88(7):3196–3201.

33. Kahaly G, Olshausen KV, Mohr-Kahaly S, Erbel R, Boor S, Beyer J, Meyer J. Arrhythmia profile in acromegaly. Eur Heart J 1992; 13(1):51–56.

34. Jenkins PJ, Sohaib SA, Akker S, Phillips RR, Spillane K, Wass JA, Monson JP, Grossman AB, Besser GM, Reznek RH. The pathology of median neuropathy in acromegaly. Ann Intern Med 2000; 133(3):197–201.

35. Jamal GA, Kerr DJ, McLellan AR, Weir AI, Davies DL. Generalised peripheral nerve dysfunction in acromegaly: a study by conventional and novel neurophysiological techniques. J Neurol Neurosurg Psychiatry 1987; 50(7):886–894.

36. Gasperi M, Martino E, Manetti L, Arosio M, Porretti S, Faglia G, Mariotti S, Colao AM, Lombardi G, Baldelli R, Camanni F, Liuzzi A. Prevalence of thyroid diseases in patients with acromegaly: results of an Italian multi-center study. J Endocrinol Invest 2002; 25(3):240–245.

37. Katznelson L, Kleinberg D, Vance ML, Stavrou S, Pulaski KJ, Schoenfeld DA, Hayden DL, Wright ME, Woodburn CJ, Klibanski A. Hypogonadism in patients with acromegaly: data from the multi-centre acromegaly registry pilot study. Clin Endocrinol (Oxf) 2001; 54(2):183–188.

38. Mestron A, Webb SM, Astorga R, Benito P, Catala M, Gaztambide S, Gomez JM, Halperin I, Lucas-Morante T, Moreno B, Obiols G, de Pablos P, Paramo C, Pico A, Torres E, Varela C, Vazquez JA, Zamora J, Albareda M, Gilabert M. Epidemiology, clinical characteristics, outcome, morbidity and mortality in acromegaly based on the Spanish Acromegaly Registry (Registro Espanol de Acromegalia, REA). Eur J Endocrinol 2004; 151(4):439–446.

39. Barrande G, Pittino-Lungo M, Coste J, Ponvert D, Bertagna X, Luton JP, Bertherat J. Hormonal and metabolic effects of radiotherapy in acromegaly: long-term results in 128 patients followed in a single center. J Clin Endocrinol Metab 2000; 85(10):3779–3785.

40. Baris D, Gridley G, Ron E, Weiderpass E, Mellemkjaer L, Ekbom A, Olsen JH, Baron JA, Fraumeni JF Jr. Acromegaly and cancer risk: a cohort study in Sweden and Denmark. Cancer Causes Control 2002; 13(5):395–400.

41. Renehan AG, O'Connell J, O'Halloran D, Shanahan F, Potten CS, O'dwyer ST, Shalet SM. Acromegaly and colorectal cancer: a comprehensive review of epidemiology, biological mechanisms, and clinical implications. Horm Metab Res 2003; 35(11–12):712–725.

42. Freda PU, Reyes CM, Nuruzzaman AT, Sundeen RE, Bruce JN. Basal and glucose-suppressed GH levels less than 1 microg/L in newly diagnosed acromegaly. Pituitary 2003; 6(4):175–180.

43. Levitt NS, Ratanjee BD, Abrahamson MJ. Do "so-called" normal growth hormone concentrations (2–5 micrograms/L) indicate cure in acromegaly? Horm Metab Res 1995; 27(4):185–188.

44. Dimaraki EV, Jaffe CA, Demott-Friberg R, Chandler WF, Barkan AL. Acromegaly with apparently normal GH secretion: implications for diagnosis and follow-up. J Clin Endocrinol Metab 2002; 87(8):3537–3542.

45. Barkan AL, Beitins IZ, Kelch RP. Plasma insulin-like growth factor-I/somatomedin-C in acromegaly: correlation with the degree of growth hormone hypersecretion. J Clin Endocrinol Metab 1988; 67(1):69–73.

46. Clemmons DR, Van Wyk JJ, Ridgway EC, Kliman B, Kjellberg RN, Underwood LE. Evaluation of acromegaly by radioimmunoassay of somatomedin-C. N Engl J Med 1979; 301(21):1138–1142.

47. Biochemical assessment and long-term monitoring in patients with acromegaly: statement from a joint consensus conference of the Growth Hormone Research Society and the Pituitary Society. J Clin Endocrinol Metab 2004; 89(7):3099–3102.

48. Daughaday WH, Starkey RH, Saltman S, Gavin JR III, Mills-Dunlap B, Heath-Monnig E. Characterization of serum growth hormone (GH) and insulin-like growth factor I in active acromegaly with minimal elevation of serum GH. J Clin Endocrinol Metab 1987; 65(4):617–623.

49. Clemmons DR, Chihara K, Freda PU, Ho KK, Klibanski A, Melmed S, Shalet SM, Strasburger CJ, Trainer PJ, Thorner MO. Optimizing control of acromegaly: integrating a growth hormone receptor antagonist into the treatment algorithm. J Clin Endocrinol Metab 2003; 88(10):4759–4767.

50. Freda PU, Post KD, Powell JS, Wardlaw SL. Evaluation of disease status with sensitive measures of growth hormone secretion in 60 postoperative patients with acromegaly. J Clin Endocrinol Metab 1998; 83(11):3808–3816.

51. Marro B, Zouaoui A, Sahel M, Crozat N, Gerber S, Sourour N, Sag K, Marsault C. MRI of pituitary adenomas in acromegaly. Neuroradiology 1997; 39(6):394–399.

52. Lundin P, Nyman R, Burman P, Lundberg PO, Muhr C. MRI of pituitary macroadenomas with reference to hormonal activity. Neuroradiology 1992; 34(1):43–51.

53. Vezina JL, Hardy J, Yamashita M. Microadenomas hypersecreting pituitary adenomas. Arq Neuropsiquiatr 1975; 33(2):119–127.

54. Bourdelot A, Coste J, Hazebroucq V, Gaillard S, Cazabat L, Bertagna X, Bertherat J. Clinical, hormonal and magnetic resonance imaging (MRI) predictors of transsphenoidal surgery outcome in acromegaly. Eur J Endocrinol 2004; 150(6):763–771.

55. Athanassiadi K, Exarchos D, Tsagarakis S, Bellenis I. Acromegaly caused by ectopic growth hormone-releasing hormone secretion by a carcinoid bronchial tumor: a rare entity. J Thorac Cardiovasc Surg 2004; 128(4):631–632.

56. Osella G, Orlandi F, Caraci P, Ventura M, Deandreis D, Papotti M, Bongio-
    vanni M, Angeli A, Terzolo M. Acromegaly due to ectopic secretion of
    GHRH by bronchial carcinoid in a patient with empty sella. J Endocrinol
    Invest 2003; 26(2):163–169.

57. Lorcy Y, Perdu S, Sevray B, Cohen R. [Acromegaly due to ectopic GH RH
    secretion by a bronchial carcinoid tumor: a case report]. Ann Endocrinol
    (Paris) 2002; 63(6 pt 1):536–539.

58. Boix E, Pico A, Pinedo R, Aranda I, Kovacs K. Ectopic growth hormone-
    releasing hormone secretion by thymic carcinoid tumour. Clin Endocrinol
    (Oxf) 2002; 57(1):131–134.

59. Doga M, Bonadonna S, Burattin A, Giustina A. Ectopic secretion of growth
    hormone-releasing hormone (GHRH) in neuroendocrine tumors: relevant
    clinical aspects. Ann Oncol 2001; 12(suppl 2):S89–S94.

60. Ezzat S, Ezrin C, Yamashita S, Melmed S. Recurrent acromegaly resulting
    from ectopic growth hormone gene expression by a metastatic pancreatic
    tumor. Cancer 1993; 71(1):66–70.

61. Melmed S, Ziel FH, Braunstein GD, Downs T, Frohman LA. Medical man-
    agement of acromegaly due to ectopic production of growth hormone-
    releasing hormone by a carcinoid tumor. J Clin Endocrinol Metab 1988;
    67(2):395–399.

62. Melmed S, Ezrin C, Kovacs K, Goodman RS, Frohman LA. Acromegaly due
    to secretion of growth hormone by an ectopic pancreatic islet-cell tumor. N
    Engl J Med 1985; 312(1):9–17.

63. Mitsuya K, Nakasu Y, Nioka H, Nakasu S. Ectopic growth hormone-
    releasing adenoma in the cavernous sinus—case report. Neurol Med Chir
    (Tokyo) 2004; 44(7):380–385.

64. Morel O, Giraud P, Bernier MO, Le Jeune JJ, Rohmer V, Jallet P. Ectopic acro-
    megaly: localization of the pituitary growth hormone-releasing hormone
    producing tumor by In-111 pentetreotide scintigraphy and report of two
    cases. Clin Nucl Med 2004; 29(12):841–843.

65. Hofland LJ, Lamberts SW, van Hagen PM, Reubi JC, Schaeffer J, Waaijers M,
    van Koetsveld PM, Srinivasan A, Krenning EP, Breeman WA. Crucial role
    for somatostatin receptor subtype 2 in determining the uptake of [111 In-
    DTPA-D-Phe1]octreotide in somatostatin receptor-positive organs. J Nucl
    Med 2003; 44(8):1315–1321.

Section III

TREATMENT

5

Surgery

INTRODUCTION

As described in Chapter 1, neurosurgery has long been an effective treatment for acromegaly. From the 1960s onward, pituitary surgery has benefited from the introduction of televisual and radiological imaging technologies, while miniaturization of instruments has allowed selective tumor resection that spares normal pituitary tissue. At present, advances in endoscopic technology are being integrated into the standard neurosurgical approaches to pituitary tumors. Given the high level of technical skill required, it comes as no surprise that outcomes from pituitary surgery are best with neurosurgeons who focus on pituitary surgery and as well as other procedures involving the pituitary gland (1,2). This chapter briefly reviews some of the technical approaches used to reach and resect pituitary tumors and discusses the outcomes achieved in large published patient series.

TECHNICAL APPROACHES TO PITUITARY SURGERY

The two main approaches to pituitary adenomas are via the transsphenoidal and the transcranial routes, with the latter being used in the case of difficult tumors with significant suprasellar or parasellar extension. Refinements and adaptations of both major approaches have been used to reach the skull base, cavernous sinuses, and other extra-pituitary sites, some of which are used to resect infiltrating or highly extensive tumors (3,4). Other, less commonly used approaches are described in the specialist literature (5,6).

Transsphenoidal Surgery

A surgeon's view of the transsphenoidal resection of a pituitary adenoma is illustrated in the series of photographs in Figure 1. The initial incision can be made sublabially, as shown in Figure 1A, or alternatively an endonasal entry may be used. Following a sublabial incision, the nasal mucosa are raised and a submucosal dissection undertaken. The cartilaginous nasal septum is resected and a speculum is used to keep the operative route clear (Fig. 1B–D). The sphenoid sinus floor is reached and opened and the sella turcica is entered. An incision is made in the dura lining the sella turcica, thus exposing the pituitary gland itself (Fig. 1E–F). Using the preoperative MRI results and intraoperative exploration, the pituitary adenoma is identified and resected away using microcurettes and other specially designed tools (Fig. 1G–H). The cavity remaining after tumor resection can be inspected using angled mirrored instruments, or, as is increasingly done, using an appropriate neurosurgical endoscope. In the case of larger adenomas, the angled view provided by an endoscope can be useful for detecting remaining tumor deposits after the main tumor body has been resected. If a cerebrospinal fluid (CSF) leak is noted at the end of surgery, this can be closed using a fat and fascia lata graft from the patient's thigh (7). The endonasal transsphenoidal approach has some benefits over the sublabial transsphenoidal approach in that the former is technically easier and is associated with lower post-operative pain (7).

Transcranial Surgery

As discussed in Chapter 1, from the late 1920s onward, Cushing favored the transcranial approach to pituitary lesions. For decades, barring a few notable exceptions, the rest of neurosurgery followed Cushing's lead. However, the reintroduction and refinement of transsphenoidal surgery by Hirsch, Dott, Guiot, and Hardy has not meant that transcranial pituitary surgery has been abandoned. In cases where tumors are suprasellar and invasive in nature or are otherwise unamenable to transsphenoidal surgery, a pterional or subfrontal transcranial operation may be undertaken. In both of these techniques, the tumor is reached via retraction of the brain and resection is performed in close relation to the optic nerves and carotids (pterional) and the olfactory tracts (subfrontal).

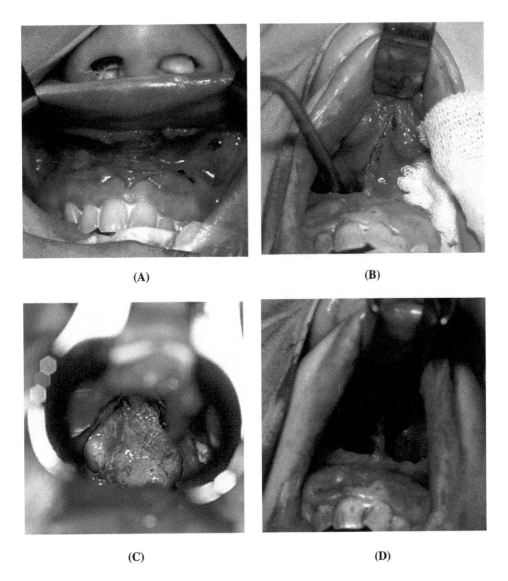

Figure 1
Transsphenoidal resection of a pituitary adenoma. In this series of images,
the initial incision is made sublabially (**A**). As shown in (**B–D**), submucosal
dissection is undertaken, the cartilaginous nasal septum is resected, and
a speculum is inserted to open and maintain the operative route. Thereafter,
the floor of the sphenoid sinus is identified and opened, and the floor of the
sella turcica is entered. After the dural lining is incised, the pituitary gland
itself is encountered (**E,F**), and the pituitary adenoma is identified and
resected (**G,H**). (*Continued*)
Source: A. Beckers and A. Stevenaert

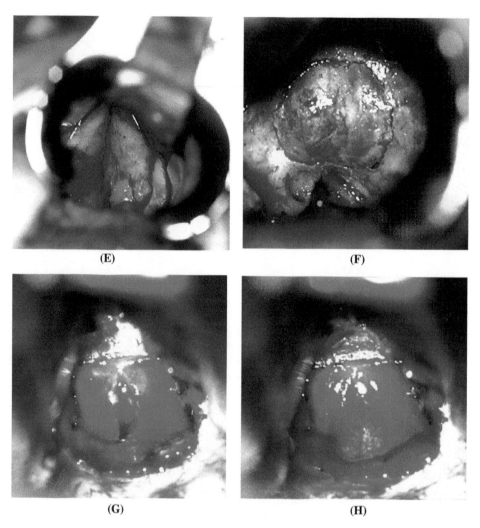

(E)   (F)

(G)   (H)

Figure 1
(*Continued*)

PREOPERATIVE MANAGEMENT

The workup of a patient before pituitary surgery should include adequate MRI imaging for identification of tumor dimensions and extension, testing of all pituitary hormonal axes, and assessment for the presence of end-organ disease, particularly in the cardiorespiratory system. Since the advent of somatostatin analog therapy for acromegaly, many patients have received preoperative treatment in order to improve their overall physical condition (8). Furthermore, a moderate degree of tumor shrinkage can occur with somatostatin analog therapy (9), which has been reported to aid tumor resection in some (8,10,11), but not all, series (12,13).

OUTCOMES OF SURGICAL TREATMENT OF ACROMEGALY

The aims of pituitary surgery for acromegaly are the total resection of the tumor or, if this is not possible, the removal of the maximum amount of tumor that is safely feasible, the preservation of healthy pituitary tissue, and the restoration of normal hormonal secretion. The success of surgery in terms of "curing" acromegaly depends on a number of factors. Primary among these is the way hormonal control is defined, which has evolved significantly over time. Earlier studies took a relatively broad definition of growth hormone (GH) control to assess the success rate of surgical series in acromegaly. A basal GH of less than 5 μg/L was considered as "controlled" acromegaly in many studies, which gave an overall surgical control rate of 65% when micro- and macroadenomas were pooled (14–19). A move toward more stringent control criteria began in the 1990s, when studies such as that of Sheaves et al. (20) demonstrated that postoperative control of acromegaly fell from 75% overall to only 42% when the basal nonsuppressed GH cut-off was lowered from 10 to 2.5 μg/L. In a large series ($n = 396$), Fahlbusch et al. (21) noted that only 58% of patients were controlled using a cut-off GH of <2 μg/L post Oral Glucose Tolerance Test (OGTT). More recent studies have employed even stricter hormonal control criteria, including a normalized IGF-I and/or a GH <1μg/L post OGTT. Using these criteria, Swearingen et al. (22) reported a cure/remission rate of 57%, which was similar to the results obtained in series reported by Freda et al. (61%) (23) and De et al. (63%) (24). Biermasz et al. (25) reported that normal post-OGTT GH and insulin-like growth factor-I (IGF-I) were present in 37% of patients after 10 years of follow-up. Recent series have reported disease control rates of 64% (United States) and 55% (Japan) 5 and 7 years after surgery, respectively, using normalized age- and sex-matched IGF-I as the control criteria (26,27). Kreutzer et al. (28) reported a higher post-operative IGF-I control rate of 70.2% in a series of 57 acromegalic patients after 1–7 years of follow-up.

Surgical cure rates in acromegaly are higher in microadenomas and contained macroadenomas (70–85%) than in extensive macroadenomas (20–50%) or invasive tumors; predictors of a poor post-operative outcome in terms of disease control in acromegaly include tumor extension or invasion, incomplete tumor resection, a high preoperative GH level, and young age at diagnosis (28–34). Low (i.e., controlled) GH in the immediate post-operative period and GH control during the first 6 weeks after surgery are predictive of long-term remission in acromegaly (27,28). It is now well recognized that surgical outcome in acromegaly is better when surgery is performed by a dedicated pituitary neurosurgeon. Ahmed et al.

(2) noted that as the experience of a dedicated pituitary surgeon increased over time, this led to a concomitant improvement in hormonal control. Gittoes and colleagues (1) noted an improvement in acromegaly outcome when pituitary management was changed from being divided among seven surgeons to just one. They reported a significant rise in the cure rate for acromegaly from 33% to 64% during this time, while microadenoma and macroadenoma cure rates rose from 54% to 86% and from 30% to 52%, respectively (1). De et al. (24) recently compared the progression in post-operative success rates over a three-decade period in Wales, during which time the responsibility for neurosurgical care of pituitary adenomas changed from the otorhinology department to a dedicated pituitary surgeon. They reported that the remission rate for acromegaly was significantly higher under the surgeon's management (76%) than during the otorhinology care era (54–63%).

REPEAT SURGERY

The necessity for a second surgical intervention may arise due to recurrence of a tumor previously thought to have been fully removed or subsequent growth of an unresectable tumor remnant. The recurrence rate for acromegaly in surgical series is less than 10% (24,35,36). Results for repeat surgery are less favorable than for initial procedures, but benefits may be achieved in terms of hormonal levels and symptom severity; disease control may be possible with adjuvant radiotherapy or medical therapy. Hardy's group in Montreal reported a series of 16 acromegalic patients who underwent recurrent surgery for progressing persistent acromegaly (11 patients), visual symptoms (4 patients), and disease recurrence (1 patient) (37). The criteria for cure was a basal GH of $<5\,\mu g/L$ and suppression of GH to $<2\,\mu g/L$ post OGTT. Following the second intervention, three patients were in remission for 2–20 years, two had a basal GH $<5\,\mu g/L$ but an abnormal OGTT value, and GH levels fell by $>50\%$ in 11 patients. As would be expected in a series of patients with severe disease, adverse events were relatively frequent, with nearly two-thirds of patients developing new pituitary hormone deficits.

Kurosaki summarized the experience of a Japanese group with second surgery for 22 patients with residual or recurring acromegaly using a transnasal approach (38). Sixteen patients had resectable tumors and six had nonresectable invasive tumors. Intraoperative GH levels were normalized initially in 56% of patients with resectable tumors, and in four others further resection controlled GH. All of these patients remained in remission during a 4-year follow-up period. In summary, repeat surgery to debulk invasive or unresectable tumors is a potentially useful step even if surgical cure is not possible.

ADVERSE EVENTS

In large centers, the mortality rate following pituitary surgery for acromegaly is low at 0–1% (29,36,39). Excluding anterior hypopituitarism, the complication rate for initial surgery has been estimated at 10–15%, and is composed of early and late complications (24,29). Early complications include hemorrhage, infection, and meningitis, while olfactory nerve damage can lead to loss of the sense of smell. Diabetes insipidus and CSF rhinorrhea may occur on a temporary or permanent basis. Hypopituitarism occurs at a variable rate post-operatively in acromegaly, with rates of less than 5% up to 30% reported in the literature, although the true figure is probably nearer the latter rate (20,24,35,40,41).

REFERENCES

1. Gittoes NJ, Sheppard MC, Johnson AP, Stewart PM. Outcome of surgery for acromegaly—the experience of a dedicated pituitary surgeon. QJM 1999; 92(12):741–745.

2. Ahmed S, Elsheikh M, Stratton IM, Page RC, Adams CB, Wass JA. Outcome of transphenoidal surgery for acromegaly and its relationship to surgical experience. Clin Endocrinol (Oxf) 1999; 50(5):561–567.

3. Couldwell WT, Weiss MH, Rabb C, Liu JK, Apfelbaum RI, Fukushima T. Variations on the standard transsphenoidal approach to the sellar region, with emphasis on the extended approaches and parasellar approaches: surgical experience in 105 cases. Neurosurgery 2004; 55(3):539–547.

4. Liu JK, Weiss MH, Couldwell WT. Surgical approaches to pituitary tumors. Neurosurg Clin N Am 2003; 14(1):93–107.

5. Sabit I, Schaefer SD, Couldwell WT. Modified infratemporal fossa approach via lateral transantral maxillotomy: a microsurgical model. Surg Neurol 2002; 58(1):21–31.

6. Karci B, Oner K, Gunhan O, Ovul I, Bilgen C. Nasomaxillary osteotomy in lesions of the central compartment of the middle cranial base. Rhinology 2001; 39(3):160–165.

7. Couldwell WT. Transsphenoidal and transcranial surgery for pituitary adenomas. J Neurooncol 2004; 69(1–3):237–256.

8. Colao A, Ferone D, Cappabianca P, Del Basso de Caro ML, Marzullo P, Monticelli A, Alfieri A, Merola B, Cali A, de Divitiis E, Lombardi G. Effect of octreotide pretreatment on surgical outcome in acromegaly. J Clin Endocrinol Metab 1997; 82(10):3308–3314.

9. Plockinger U, Reichel M, Fett U, Saeger W, Quabbe HJ. Preoperative octreotide treatment of growth hormone-secreting and clinically nonfunctioning pituitary macroadenomas: effect on tumor volume and lack of correlation with immunohistochemistry and somatostatin receptor scintigraphy. J Clin Endocrinol Metab 1994; 79(5):1416–1423.

10. Stevenaert A, Beckers A. Presurgical Octreotide: treatment in acromegaly. Metabolism 1996; 45(8) (suppl):72–74.

11. Barkan AL, Lloyd RV, Chandler WF, Hatfield MK, Gebarski SS, Kelch RP, Beitins IZ. Preoperative treatment of acromegaly with long-acting somatostatin analog SMS 201-995: shrinkage of invasive pituitary macroadenomas and improved surgical remission rate. J Clin Endocrinol Metab 1988; 67(5):1040–1048.

12. Kristof RA, Stoffel-Wagner B, Klingmuller D, Schramm J. Does octreotide treatment improve the surgical results of macro-adenomas in acromegaly? A randomized study. Acta Neurochir (Wien) 1999; 141(4):399–405.

13. Lucas-Morante T, Garcia-Uria J, Estrada J, Saucedo G, Cabello A, Alcaniz J, Barcelo B. Treatment of invasive growth hormone pituitary adenomas with long-acting somatostatin analog SMS 201-995 before transsphenoidal surgery. J Neurosurg 1994; 81(1):10–14.

14. Teasdale GM, Hay ID, Beasttall GH, McCruden DC, Thomson JA, Davies DL, Grossart KW, Ratcliffe JG. Cryosurgery or microsurgery in the management of acromegaly. JAMA 1982; 247(9):1289–1291.

15. Ross DA, Wilson CB. Results of transsphenoidal microsurgery for growth hormone-secreting pituitary adenoma in a series of 214 patients. J Neurosurg 1988; 68(6):854–867.

16. Tindall GT, Oyesiku NM, Watts NB, Clark RV, Christy JH, Adams DA. Transsphenoidal adenomectomy for growth hormone-secreting pituitary adenomas in acromegaly: outcome analysis and determinants of failure. J Neurosurg 1993; 78(2):205–215.

17. Davis DH, Laws ER Jr, Ilstrup DM, Speed JK, Caruso M, Shaw EG, Abboud CF, Scheithauer BW, Root LM, Schleck C. Results of surgical treatment for growth hormone-secreting pituitary adenomas. J Neurosurg 1993; 79(1):70–75.

18. Fahlbusch R, Honegger J, Buchfelder M. Surgical management of acromegaly. Endocrinol Metab Clin North Am 1992; 21(3):669–692.

19. Grisoli F, Leclercq T, Jaquet P, Guibout M, Winteler JP, Hassoun J, Vincentelli F. Transsphenoidal surgery for acromegaly—long-term results in 100 patients. Surg Neurol 1985; 23(5):513–519.

20. Sheaves R, Jenkins P, Blackburn P, Huneidi AH, Afshar F, Medbak S, Grossman AB, Besser GM, Wass JA. Outcome of transsphenoidal surgery for acromegaly using strict criteria for surgical cure. Clin Endocrinol (Oxf) 1996; 45(4):407–413.

21. Fahlbusch R, Honegger J, Buchfelder M. Evidence supporting surgery as treatment of choice for acromegaly. J Endocrinol 1997; 155(suppl 1):S53–S55.

22. Swearingen B, Barker FG, Katznelson L, Biller BM, Grinspoon S, Klibanski A, Moayeri N, Black PM, Zervas NT. Long-term mortality after transsphenoidal surgery and adjunctive therapy for acromegaly. J Clin Endocrinol Metab 1998; 83(10):3419–3426.

23. Freda PU, Wardlaw SL, Post KD. Long-term endocrinological follow-up evaluation in 115 patients who underwent transsphenoidal surgery for acromegaly. J Neurosurg 1998; 89(3):353–358.

24. De P, Rees DA, Davies N, John R, Neal J, Mills RG, Vafidis J, Davies JS, Scanlon MF. Transsphenoidal surgery for acromegaly in wales: results based on stringent criteria of remission. J Clin Endocrinol Metab 2003; 88(8): 3567–3572.

25. Biermasz NR, van Dulken H, Roelfsema F. Ten-year follow-up results of transsphenoidal microsurgery in acromegaly. J Clin Endocrinol Metab 2000; 85(12):4596–4602.

26. Takahashi JA, Shimatsu A, Nakao K, Hashimoto N. Early postoperative indicators of late outcome in acromegalic patients. Clin Endocrinol (Oxf) 2004; 60(3):366–374.

27. Krieger MD, Couldwell WT, Weiss MH. Assessment of long-term remission of acromegaly following surgery. J Neurosurg 2003; 98(4):719–724.

28. Kreutzer J, Vance ML, Lopes MB, Laws ER Jr. Surgical management of GH-secreting pituitary adenomas: an outcome study using modern remission criteria. J Clin Endocrinol Metab 2001; 86(9):4072–4077.

29. Minniti G, Jaffrain-Rea ML, Esposito V, Santoro A, Tamburrano G, Cantore G. Evolving criteria for post-operative biochemical remission of acromegaly: can we achieve a definitive cure? An audit of surgical results on a large series and a review of the literature. Endocr Relat Cancer 2003; 10(4):611–619.

30. Esposito V, Santoro A, Minniti G, Salvati M, Innocenzi G, Lanzetta G, Cantore G. Transsphenoidal adenomectomy for GH-, PRL- and ACTH-secreting pituitary tumours: outcome analysis in a series of 125 patients. Neurol Sci 2004; 25(5):251–256.

31. Shimon I, Cohen ZR, Ram Z, Hadani M. Transsphenoidal surgery for acromegaly: endocrinological follow-up of 98 patients. Neurosurgery 2001; 48(6):1239–1243.

32. Kaltsas GA, Isidori AM, Florakis D, Trainer PJ, Camacho-Hubner C, Afshar F, Sabin I, Jenkins JP, Chew SL, Monson JP, Besser GM, Grossman AB. Predictors of the outcome of surgical treatment in acromegaly and the value of the mean growth hormone day curve in assessing postoperative disease activity. J Clin Endocrinol Metab 2001; 86(4):1645–1652.

33. Trepp R, Stettler C, Zwahlen M, Seiler R, Diem P, Christ ER. Treatment outcomes and mortality of 94 patients with acromegaly. Acta Neurochir (Wien) 2005; 10.1007/s00701–004–0466–2.

34. Bourdelot A, Coste J, Hazebroucq V, Gaillard S, Cazabat L, Bertagna X, Bertherat J. Clinical, hormonal and magnetic resonance imaging (MRI) predictors of transsphenoidal surgery outcome in acromegaly. Eur J Endocrinol 2004; 150(6):763–771.

35. Abosch A, Tyrrell JB, Lamborn KR, Hannegan LT, Applebury CB, Wilson CB. Transsphenoidal microsurgery for growth hormone-secreting pituitary adenomas: initial outcome and long-term results. J Clin Endocrinol Metab 1998; 83(10):3411–3418.

36. Beauregard C, Truong U, Hardy J, Serri O. Long-term outcome and mortality after transsphenoidal adenomectomy for acromegaly. Clin Endocrinol (Oxf) 2003; 58(1):86–91.

37. Long H, Beauregard H, Somma M, Comtois R, Serri O, Hardy J. Surgical
     outcome after repeated transsphenoidal surgery in acromegaly. J Neurosurg
     1996; 85(2):239–247.

38. Kurosaki M, Luedecke DK, Abe T. Effectiveness of secondary transnasal
     surgery in GH-secreting pituitary macroadenomas. Endocr J 2003; 50(5):
     635–642.

39. Nomikos P, Ladar C, Fahlbusch R, Buchfelder M. Impact of primary surgery
     on pituitary function in patients with non-functioning pituitary adenomas—
     a study on 721 patients. Acta Neurochir (Wien) 2004; 146(1):27–35.

40. Inder WJ, Espiner EA, MacFarlane MR. Outcome from surgical management
     of secretory pituitary adenomas in Christchurch, New Zealand. Intern Med J
     2003; 33(4):168–173.

41. van Lindert E, Hey O, Boecher-Schwarz H, Perneczky A. Treatment results
     of acromegaly as analyzed by different criteria. Acta Neurochir (Wien) 1997;
     139(10):905–912.

6

Somatostatin Analogs

BACKGROUND

Soon after the identification of somatostatin as an inhibitor of growth hormone (GH) secretion by Guillemin's group (1), it was realized that somatostatin could be harnessed as a treatment for acromegaly (2). However, the short plasma half-life of native somatostatin, which necessitated administration by continuous infusion, limited its direct applicability to the clinical scenario. It was suggested that a long-acting analog of somatostatin could overcome this limitation (3), and a series of pharmacological programs were put in place to synthesize such a compound. This process culminated in 1982 with the development of an octapeptide somatostatin analog, octreotide (SMS 201–995), which had a plasma half-life of approximately 90 minutes and inhibited GH more potently than insulin or glucagon (Fig. 1). A variety of other somatostatin analogs followed (4,5). The development of somatostatin analogs led to a better appreciation of the nature of somatostatin receptors. There are now known to be five somatostatin receptors, of which somatostatin receptor subtypes 2 and 5 are the predominant forms found in the pituitary and GH-secreting pituitary adenomas (6). Somatostatin analogs in clinical use today (octreotide and lanreotide) are relatively specific for the subtype 2 receptor.

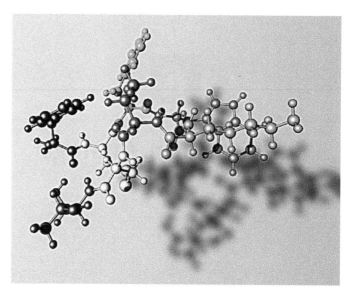

Figure 1
Three-dimensional structure of the somatostatin analog octreotide.
Source: A. Beckers and P. Petrossians. Image developed from data in Melacini G. et al. Biochemistry 1997; 36: 1233, and Berman, H. M. et al. Nucl Acid Res 2000; 28: 235–242.

SOMATOSTATIN ANALOGS IN ACROMEGALY: EARLY STUDIES

Initial studies of octreotide in acromegaly were performed in the mid 1980s by Lamberts et al. and others (7–9). These studies demonstrated that marked GH and insulin-like growth factor-I (IGF-I) (termed somatomedin-C at that time) suppression could be achieved safely over the short and long term. Larger national and international open label studies were performed that confirmed the efficacy and safety of octreotide in this regard (10,11). A prospective placebo-controlled trial was performed in the United States and Canada in which 115 acromegalic patients received octreotide three times a day for 6 months (12). Mean GH levels were decreased to less than $5\,\mu g/L$ in up to 53% of patients, while IGF-I was normalized in up to 66%. This study was continued in an open label fashion for up to 30 months and demonstrated that the suppression of GH and IGF-I achieved initially with octreotide was sustained for more than 2 years (13).

DEPOT FORMULATIONS OF SOMATOSTATIN ANALOGS

While intermittent administration of somatostatin analogs was found to be effective for the treatment of acromegaly, the inconvenience of repeated injections led to the development of long-acting depot formulations.

Octreotide long-acting repeatable (LAR) consists of octreotide-impregnated biodegradable DL-lactide-co-glycolide microspheres. After deep intramuscular injection, octreotide is released from the microspheres, and initially peaks within 1 hour, but thereafter plateaus after the first week post-administration (14–16). The peak-to-trough variations in dose following depot administration of octreotide (and other somatostatin analogs) is approximately 25%, compared with nearly ten times this amount during intermittent subcutaneous therapy. Octreotide concentrations fall gradually after day 42; thus, octreotide LAR is ideally given once a month, although some patients may tolerate longer dosage intervals (17). A slow-release formulation of lanreotide, lanreotide SR, has also been used widely. The formulation of lanreotide SR means that it is ideally given every 14 days or so (18–20). More recently, an aqueous microparticle form of lanreotide, lanreotide Autogel, has been developed and shown to be effective in the long-term control of acromegaly (21,22). The biochemical and clinical efficacies of intermittent and long-acting formulations of somatostatin analogs are broadly similar (23), but the advantage of increased patient compliance gives the long-acting formulations a practical advantage.

EFFICACY OF LONG-ACTING SOMATOSTATIN ANALOGS

Since the early 1990s, numerous large studies examining the efficacy and safety of long-acting somatostatin analogs have been performed in acromegaly. A systematic review of these data has been undertaken to determine the overall effects of long-acting somatostatin analog treatment on biochemical control in acromegaly (23). The criterion used for normalization of GH secretion was a mean/nadir GH < 2.0–$2.5\,\mu g/L$ or a post-Oral Glucose Tolerance Test (OGTT) GH concentration of $< 1.0\,\mu g/L$. For IGF-I, control was defined as normalization for the appropriate age range. In patients undergoing adjunctive somatostatin analog therapy ($n = 301$), GH control occurred in a mean of 56% of cases (range, 47–75%) treated with octreotide LAR and in 49% of patients ($n = 404$) treated with lanreotide SR (range, 14–78%). IGF-I normalization occurred in 66% (range, 41–75%) and 48% (range, 30–63%) of patients treated with octreotide LAR and lanreotide SR, respectively (Fig. 2). It should be noted that responses to somatostatin analogs are less in patients with somatostatin receptor negative tumors (24), which may explain, in part, the lack of hormonal control seen in up to one-third of patients in these clinical series.

The concept of primary medical therapy with somatostatin analogs has gained popularity in recent years (25). This is based partially on the idea that acromegalic patients who have little prospect of complete surgical resection of their pituitary adenoma could benefit from medical treatment. Data supportive of this come from a subanalysis of the North American

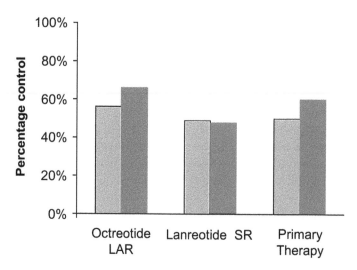

Figure 2
Rates of control of GH (gray) and IGF-I (green) during treatment with depot
somatostatin analogs. The efficacy data for primary medical therapy are derived
from studies that included patients treated with intermittent injectable and depot
forms of somatostatin analogs.
Source: Developed from data reported in Ref. 23.

Multicenter Octreotide Study noted above, in which a group of patients
who did not undergo surgery had a similar reduction in GH and IGF-I
compared to patients receiving octreotide as adjuvant therapy (26).
While patients receiving primary medical therapy with a somatostatin
analog can experience biochemical control, this is not always the case.
Petrossians et al. recently reported hormonal control rates with somatostatin analog therapy in a series of 24 acromegalic patients before and
after gross total resection or debulking of a pituitary adenoma (27). Preoperative somatostatin therapy controlled IGF-I in 45.8% of patients,
whereas in post-operative somatostatin analog treatment, this IGF-I was
normalized in 78.3%.

Freda (23) reviewed the biochemical outcome of patients receiving
primary medical therapy with somatostatin analogs (both intermittent
injectable and depot formulations of all analogs were included). GH control was achieved in 50% of patients (range, 27–77%), while IGF-I normalization occurred in 60% of cases (range, 28–90%). Taking biochemical
control results together, it appears on the surface that octreotide LAR holds
a moderate advantage over lanreotide SR. However, it should be noted
that the majority of patients in octreotide LAR trials were recruited on
the basis that they were already octreotide responders (GH suppression
following an acute subcutaneous injection of octreotide). Lanreotide SR
studies did not use this entry criterion as rigorously. Thus, caution should

be used when apportioning superiority for one depot somatostatin analog over another. Indeed, while direct comparisons indicate that octreotide LAR exhibits better biochemical control that lanreotide SR (28–30), this conclusion is not borne out in newer studies comparing lanreotide Autogel and octreotide LAR (31–33). Overall, primary medical therapy with a somatostatin analog represents a valid option for patients who are physically unsuitable for neurosurgery, particularly elderly, debilitated individuals. Some patients that are unwilling to undergo surgery may elect to receive primary medical therapy; however, if inadequate hormonal control is noted, additional treatment options should be considered, and the topic of neurosurgery may have to be re-explored.

SIGNS AND SYMPTOMS

Improvements in symptoms of acromegaly occur relatively rapidly with somatostatin analogs, often before objective evidence of regression of signs. The efficacies of depot and intermittent injectable forms of somatostatin analogs are similarly effective at controlling signs and symptoms (60–75% of patients with both therapies) (10,12,23). Headache has been noted to be particularly amenable to somatostatin analog therapy and may occur rapidly and without measurable tumor shrinkage (34); it may be that somatostatin analogs function as analgesics in this regard (35–37). Somatostatin analogs have been reported to have a variety of other effects on pathological changes associated with acromegaly; these are enumerated in Table 1.

TUMOR SHRINKAGE

Somatostatin analog therapy can produce variable shrinkage of pituitary tumors in acromegaly (10,38). The nature of this shrinkage is still not well understood, as therapy is associated with a wide variety of morphological changes in subsequently resected tumor tissue (39). Fibrosis, changes in secretory granule size and number, and overall cell size shrinkage have been reported at a histological level in GH-secreting pituitary adenomas after octreotide therapy. Apoptosis or other cytotoxic indices are not found (40,41).

A systematic review of the effects of short-acting and long-acting somatostatin analogs on tumor shrinkage was recently published (42). In 22 studies of subcutaneous intermittent octreotide, 45% of patients had tumor shrinkage, while in patients treated with octreotide LAR the overall tumor shrinkage response rate was 57%. In more than 900 patients treated with any type or formulation of somatostatin analog considered together, tumor shrinkage occurred in 42% of cases overall, in 52% of cases receiving primary medical therapy, and in 21% of patients receiving adjunctive therapy (42). The degree of shrinkage reported during somatostatin analog therapy varies widely, but overall is modest in nature and occurs in about one-third of patients overall (23). In a meta-analyses of clinical trials of somatostatin analogs, Freda reported that 12% of patients experienced $< 20\%$ shrinkage, 80% experienced 20–50% shrinkage, and $< 1\%$ experienced tumor shrinkage in excess of 50% (23). While figures for tumor shrinkage are somewhat higher for patients that received primary medical therapy with somatostatin analogs, many patients from these trials were preselected as being somatostatin-analog sensitive.

The effect of somatostatin analogs on tumor size may be temporary, as tumor re-expansion has been reported following withdrawal of somatostatin analog therapy (12,14,43–45). Presurgical somatostatin analog therapy has been employed on a regular basis at some centers for many years (38). While this treatment may make subsequent resection somewhat easier, the main reason for treating acromegalic patients preoperatively is to improve physical status and reduce anesthetic risk (46).

It is seldom appreciated, but a small number of aggressive tumors in acromegaly may continue to grow on somatostatin analog therapy. This rate of tumor progression on somatostatin analog therapy has been estimated as 2.2% (20/921 cases) (42).

ADVERSE EVENTS

Somatostatin inhibits a broad range of gastrointestinal and pancreatic hormones, modulates hepatic and intestinal blood flow, and decreases gut motility (47). Transient abdominal discomfort, bloating, and steatorrhea may complicate somatostatin analog therapy of acromegaly, but are usually mild. Inhibition of biliary motility and alterations in the components of bile increase the risk of biliary sludge and gallstones in patients receiving somatostatin analogs (48–52). About 20% of patients receiving octreotide develop new biliary sludge or gallstones (53). Ideally, patients should have a gallbladder ultrasound before initiating somatostatin analog therapy and the development of symptomatic gallstones ($< 1\%$ of cases) should be managed as in sporadic cases.

Inhibition of insulin by somatostatin analogs can further worsen carbohydrate metabolism in acromegaly, particularly in the post-prandial state. In the largest specific study of glucose tolerance during somatostatin analog treatment of acromegaly, it was shown that in the 55 patients with normal glucose tolerance before octreotide therapy, 20% developed impaired glucose tolerance and a further 29% became diabetic. The main cause of the impaired glucose tolerance was decreased insulin secretion (54). Acromegalic patients should undergo regular surveillance for impaired glucose tolerance/diabetes while receiving somatostatin analog therapy.

Table 1

Other Effects of Somatostatin Analogs in Acromegaly

Cardiovascular
Reduced left ventricular mass (55,56)
Improved left ventricular function at rest (56,57) and in response to exercise (56,58)
Decreased cardiac conduction defects/arrhythmias (59,60)
Improvement in cardiac failure (61)

Pain
Analgesic effect on acromegaly-associated headache (62–66)

Musculoskeletal
Reduced thickness of weight-bearing and non-weight-bearing joints (67)

Respiratory
Decreased tongue volume (68,69)
Improvement in severity of obstructive sleep apnea (68–72)

REFERENCES

1. Brazeau P, Guillemin R. Editorial: Somatostatin: newcomer from the hypothalamus. N Engl J Med 1974; 290(17):963–964.

2. Hall R, Besser GM, Schally AV, Coy DH, Evered D, Goldie DJ, Kastin AJ, McNeilly AS, Mortimer CH, Phenekos C, Tunbridge WM, Weightman D. Action of growth-hormone-release inhibitory hormone in healthy men and in acromegaly. Lancet 1973; 2(7829):581–584.

3. Evered DC, Gomez-Pan A, Tunbridge WM, Hall R, Lind T, Besser GM, Mortimer CH, Thorner MO, Schally AV, Kastin AJ, Coy DH. Letter: Analogues of growth-hormone release-inhibiting hormone. Lancet 1975; 1(7918):1250.

4. Wajchenberg BL, Cesar FP, Leme CE, Borghi VC, Souza VC, Souza IT, Neto DG, Germek OA, Coy DH, Comaru-Schally AM. Dissociated effects of somatostatin analogs on arginine-induced insulin, glucagon and growth hormone release in acromegalic patients. Horm Metab Res 1983; 15(10):471–474.

5. Heron I, Thomas F, Dero M, Poutrain JR, Henane S, Catus F, Kuhn JM. [Treatment of acromegaly with sustained-release lanreotide. A new somatostatin analog]. Presse Med 1993; 22(11):526–531.

6. Reubi JC, Kvols L, Krenning E, Lamberts SW. Distribution of somatostatin receptors in normal and tumor tissue. Metabolism 1990; 39(9) (suppl 2):78–81.

7. Lamberts SW, Uitterlinden P, Verschoor L, van Dongen KJ, Del Pozo E. Long-term treatment of acromegaly with the somatostatin analogue SMS 201-995. N Engl J Med 1985; 19:313(25):1576–1580.

8. Lamberts SW, Oosterom R, Neufeld M, Del Pozo E. The somatostatin analog SMS 201-995 induces long-acting inhibition of growth hormone secretion without rebound hypersecretion in acromegalic patients. J Clin Endocrinol Metab 1985; 60(6):1161–1165.

9. Horikawa R, Takano K, Hizuka N, Asakawa K, Shibasaki T, Masuda A, Shizume K. Effect of a single administration of somatostatin analogue

(SMS 201-995) on GH, TSH and insulin secretion in patients with acromegaly. Endocrinol Jpn 1986; 33(6):743–749.

10. Vance ML, Harris AG. Long-term treatment of 189 acromegalic patients with the somatostatin analog octreotide. Results of the International Multicenter Acromegaly Study Group. Arch Intern Med 1991; 151(8):1573–1578.

11. Sassolas G, Harris AG, James-Deidier A. Long term effect of incremental doses of the somatostatin analog SMS 201-995 in 58 acromegalic patients. French SMS 201-995 approximately equal to Acromegaly Study Group. J Clin Endocrinol Metab 1990; 71(2):391–397.

12. Ezzat S, Snyder PJ, Young WF, Boyajy LD, Newman C, Klibanski A, Molitch ME, Boyd AE, Sheeler L, Cook DM. Octreotide treatment of acromegaly. A randomized, multicenter study. Ann Intern Med 1992; 117(9): 711–718.

13. Newman CB, Melmed S, Snyder PJ, Young WF, Boyajy LD, Levy R, Stewart WN, Klibanski A, Molitch ME, Gagel RF. Safety and efficacy of long-term octreotide therapy of acromegaly: results of a multicenter trial in 103 patients—a clinical research center study. J Clin Endocrinol Metab 1995; 80(9):2768–2775.

14. Flogstad AK, Halse J, Haldorsen T, Lancranjan I, Marbach P, Bruns C, Jervell J. Sandostatin LAR in acromegalic patients: a dose-range study. J Clin Endocrinol Metab 1995; 80(12):3601–3607.

15. Stewart PM, Kane KF, Stewart SE, Lancranjan I, Sheppard MC. Depot long-acting somatostatin analog (Sandostatin-LAR) is an effective treatment for acromegaly. J Clin Endocrinol Metab 1995; 80(11):3267–3272.

16. Grass P, Marbach P, Bruns C, Lancranjan I. Sandostatin LAR (microencapsulated octreotide acetate) in acromegaly: pharmacokinetic and pharmacodynamic relationships. Metabolism 1996; 45(8) (suppl 1):27–30.

17. Turner HE, Thornton-Jones VA, Wass JA. Systematic dose-extension of octreotide LAR: the importance of individual tailoring of treatment in patients with acromegaly. Clin Endocrinol (Oxf) 2004; 61(2):224–231.

18. Morange I, De Boisvilliers F, Chanson P, Lucas B, DeWailly D, Catus F, Thomas F, Jaquet P. Slow release lanreotide treatment in acromegalic patients previously normalized by octreotide. J Clin Endocrinol Metab 1994; 79(1):145–151.

19. Soule S, Conway G, Hatfield A, Jacobs H. Effectiveness and tolerability of slow release lanreotide treatment in active acromegaly: six-month report on an Italian multicentre study. J Clin Endocrinol Metab 1996; 81(12): 4502–4503.

20. Giusti M, Ciccarelli E, Dallabonzana D, Delitala G, Faglia G, Liuzzi A, Gussoni G, Giordano DG. Clinical results of long-term slow-release lanreotide treatment of acromegaly. Eur J Clin Invest 1997; 27(4):277–284.

21. Caron P, Beckers A, Cullen DR, Goth MI, Gutt B, Laurberg P, Pico AM, Valimaki M, Zgliczynski W. Efficacy of the new long-acting formulation of lanreotide (lanreotide Autogel) in the management of acromegaly. J Clin Endocrinol Metab 2002; 87(1):99–104.

22. Caron P, Bex M, Cullen DR, Feldt-Rasmussen U, Pico Alfonso AM, Pynka S, Racz K, Schopohl J, Tabarin A, Valimaki MJ. One-year follow-up of patients with acromegaly treated with fixed or titrated doses of lanreotide Autogel. Clin Endocrinol (Oxf) 2004; 60(6):734–740.

23. Freda PU. Somatostatin analogs in acromegaly. J Clin Endocrinol Metab 2002; 87(7):3013–3018.

24. Park C, Yang I, Woo J, Kim S, Kim J, Kim Y, Sohn S, Kim E, Lee M, Park H, Jung J, Park S. Somatostatin (SRIF) receptor subtype 2 and 5 gene expression in growth hormone-secreting pituitary adenomas: the relationship with endogenous srif activity and response to octreotide. Endocr J 2004; 51(2): 227–236.

25. Sheppard MC. Primary medical therapy for acromegaly. Clin Endocrinol (Oxf) 2003; 58(4):387–399.

26. Newman CB, Melmed S, George A, Torigian D, Duhaney M, Snyder P, Young W, Klibanski A, Molitch ME, Gagel R, Sheeler L, Cook D, Malarkey W, Jackson I, Vance ML, Barkan A, Frohman L, Kleinberg DL. Octreotide as primary therapy for acromegaly. J Clin Endocrinol Metab 1998; 83(9): 3034–3040.

27. Petrossians P, Borges-Martins L, Espinoza C, Daly A, Betea D, Valdes-Socin H, Stevenaert A, Chanson P, Beckers A. Gross total resection or debulking of pituitary adenomas improves hormonal control of acromegaly by somatostatin analogs. Eur J Endocrinol 2005; 152(1):61–66.

28. Cozzi R, Dallabonzana D, Attanasio R, Barausse M, Oppizzi G. A comparison between octreotide-LAR and lanreotide-SR in the chronic treatment of acromegaly. Eur J Endocrinol 1999; 141(3):267–271.

29. Kendall-Taylor P, Miller M, Gebbie J, Turner S, al Maskari M. Long-acting octreotide LAR compared with lanreotide SR in the treatment of acromegaly. Pituitary 2000; 3(2):61–65.

30. Chanson P, Boerlin V, Ajzenberg C, Bachelot Y, Benito P, Bringer J, Caron P, Charbonnel B, Cortet C, Delemer B, Escobar-Jimenez F, Foubert L, Gaztambide S, Jockenhoevel F, Kuhn JM, Leclere J, Lorcy Y, Perlemuter L, Prestele H, Roger P, Rohmer V, Santen R, Sassolas G, Scherbaum WA, Schopohl J, Torres E, Varela C, Villamil F, Webb SM. Comparison of octreotide acetate LAR and lanreotide SR in patients with acromegaly. Clin Endocrinol (Oxf) 2000; 53(5):577–586.

31. Alexopoulou O, Abrams P, Verhelst J, Poppe K, Velkeniers B, Abs R, Maiter D. Efficacy and tolerability of lanreotide Autogel therapy in acromegalic patients previously treated with octreotide LAR. Eur J Endocrinol 2004; 151(3):317–324.

32. van Thiel SW, Romijn JA, Biermasz NR, Ballieux BE, Frolich M, Smit JW, Corssmit EP, Roelfsema F, Pereira AM. Octreotide long-acting repeatable and lanreotide Autogel are equally effective in controlling growth hormone secretion in acromegalic patients. Eur J Endocrinol 2004; 150(4):489–495.

33. Ashwell SG, Bevan JS, Edwards OM, Harris MM, Holmes C, Middleton MA, James RA. The efficacy and safety of lanreotide Autogel in patients with

acromegaly previously treated with octreotide LAR. Eur J Endocrinol 2004; 150(4):473–480.

34. Levy MJ, Bejon P, Barakat M, Goadsby PJ, Meeran K. Acromegaly: a unique human headache model. Headache 2003; 43(7):794–797.

35. Donangelo I, Rodacki M, Peixoto MC, Vaisman M, Caldas NR, Gadelha MR. Dependency and analgesia related to treatment with subcutaneous octreotide in patients with growth hormone-secreting tumors. Endocr Pract 2004; 10(2):107–111.

36. Sicolo N, Martini C, Ferla S, Roggenkamp J, Vettor R, De Palo C, Federspil G. [Analgesic effect of Sandostatin (SMS 201–995) in acromegaly headache]. Minerva Endocrinol 1990; 15(1):37–42.

37. Paunovic VR, Popovic V. The development of dependence to an octapeptide somatostatin analog: contribution to the study of somatostatin analgesia. Biol Psychiatry 1989; 26(1):97–101.

38. Stevenaert A, Harris AG, Kovacs K, Beckers A. Presurgical octreotide treatment in acromegaly. Metabolism 1992; 41(9) (suppl 2):51–58.

39. Ezzat S, Kontogeorgos G, Redelmeier DA, Horvath E, Harris AG, Kovacs K. In vivo responsiveness of morphological variants of growth hormone-producing pituitary adenomas to octreotide. Eur J Endocrinol 1995; 133(6): 686–690.

40. Ezzat S, Horvath E, Harris AG, Kovacs K. Morphological effects of octreotide on growth hormone-producing pituitary adenomas. J Clin Endocrinol Metab 1994; 79(1):113–118.

41. Losa M, Ciccarelli E, Mortini P, Barzaghi R, Gaia D, Faccani G, Papotti M, Mangili F, Terreni MR, Camanni F, Giovanelli M. Effects of octreotide treatment on the proliferation and apoptotic index of GH-secreting pituitary adenomas. J Clin Endocrinol Metab 2001; 86(11):5194–5200.

42. Bevan JS. The anti-turmoral effects of somatostatin analog therapy in acromegaly. J Clin Endocrinol Metab 2005; 90(3):1856–1863.

43. Barakat S, Melmed S. Reversible shrinkage of a growth hormone-secreting pituitary adenoma by a long-acting somatostatin analogue, octreotide. Arch Intern Med 1989; 149(6):1443–1445.

44. Arosio M, Macchelli S, Rossi CM, Casati G, Biella O, Faglia G. Effects of treatment with octreotide in acromegalic patients—a multicenter Italian study. Italian Multicenter Octreotide Study Group. Eur J Endocrinol 1995; 133(4):430–439.

45. Lundin P, Eden Engstrom B, Karlsson FA, Burman P. Long-term octreotide therapy in growth hormone-secreting pituitary adenomas: evaluation with serial MR. AJNR Am J Neuroradiol 1997; 18(4):765–772.

46. Ben Shlomo A, Melmed S. Clinical review 154: The role of pharmacotherapy in perioperative management of patients with acromegaly. J Clin Endocrinol Metab 2003; 88(3):963–968.

47. Lamberts SW, van der Lely AJ, de Herder WW, Hofland LJ. Octreotide. N Engl J Med 1996; 334(4):246–254.

48. Catnach SM, Anderson JV, Fairclough PD, Trembath RC, Wilson PA, Parker E, Besser GM, Wass JA. Effect of octreotide on gall stone prevalence and gall bladder motility in acromegaly. Gut 1993; 34(2):270–273.

49. Catnach SM, Wass JA, Anderson JV, Besser M, Fairclough P, Hussaini H, Dowling H. Gall stones induced by octreotide. BMJ 1992; 305(6848):313.

50. Schmidt K, Leuschner M, Harris AG, Althoff PH, Jacobi V, Jungmann E, Schumm-Draeger PM, Rau H, Braulke C, Usadel KH. Gallstones in acromegalic patients undergoing different treatment regimens. Clin Investig 1992; 70(7):556–559.

51. Dowling RH. Review: pathogenesis of gallstones. Aliment Pharmacol Ther 2000; 14(suppl 2):39–47.

52. Veysey MJ, Thomas LA, Mallet AI, Jenkins PJ, Besser GM, Wass JA, Murphy GM, Dowling RH. Prolonged large bowel transit increases serum deoxycholic acid: a risk factor for octreotide induced gallstones. Gut 1999; 44(5):675–681.

53. Cozzi R, Attanasio R, Montini M, Pagani G, Lasio G, Lodrini S, Barausse M, Albizzi M, Dallabonzana D, Pedroncelli AM. Four-year treatment with octreotide-long-acting repeatable in 110 acromegalic patients: predictive value of short-term results? J Clin Endocrinol Metab 2003; 88(7):3090–3098.

54. Koop BL, Harris AG, Ezzat S. Effect of octreotide on glucose tolerance in acromegaly. Eur J Endocrinol 1994; 130(6):581–586.

55. Lim MJ, Barkan AL, Buda AJ. Rapid reduction of left ventricular hypertrophy in acromegaly after suppression of growth hormone hypersecretion. Ann Intern Med 1992; 117(9):719–726.

56. Colao A, Marzullo P, Ferone D, Spinelli L, Cuocolo A, Bonaduce D, Salvatore M, Boerlin V, Lancranjan I, Lombardi G. Cardiovascular effects of depot long-acting somatostatin analog Sandostatin LAR in acromegaly. J Clin Endocrinol Metab 2000; 85(9):3132–3140.

57. Gilbert J, Ketchen M, Kane P, Mason T, Baister E, Monaghan M, Barr S, Harris PE. The treatment of de novo acromegalic patients with octreotide-LAR: efficacy, tolerability and cardiovascular effects. Pituitary 2003; 6(1):11–18.

58. Colao A, Cuocolo A, Marzullo P, Nicolai E, Ferone D, Della Morte AM, Pivonello R, Salvatore M, Lombardi G. Is the acromegalic cardiomyopathy reversible? Effect of 5-year normalization of growth hormone and insulin-like growth factor I levels on cardiac performance. J Clin Endocrinol Metab 2001; 86(4):1551–1557.

59. Tachibana H, Yamaguchi H, Abe S, Sato T, Inoue S, Abe S, Yamaki M, Kubota I. Improvement of ventricular arrhythmia by octreotide treatment in acromegalic cardiomyopathy. Jpn Heart J 2003; 44(6):1027–1031.

60. Suyama K, Uchida D, Tanaka T, Saito J, Noguchi Y, Nakamura S, Tatsuno I, Saito Y, Saeki N. Octreotide improved ventricular arrhythmia in an acromegalic patient. Endocr J 2000; 47 (suppl):S73–S75.

61. Chanson P, Timsit J, Masquet C, Warnet A, Guillausseau PJ, Birman P, Harris AG, Lubetzki J. Cardiovascular effects of the somatostatin analog octreotide in acromegaly. Ann Intern Med 1990; 113(12):921–925.

62. Otsuka F, Mizobuchi S, Ogura T, Sato K, Yokoyama M, Makino H. Long-term effects of octreotide on pituitary gigantism: its analgesic action on cluster headache. Endocr J 2004; 51(5):449–452.

63. Schmidt K, Althoff PH, Harris AG, Prestele H, Schumm-Draeger PM, Usadel KH. Analgesic effect of the somatostatin analogue octreotide in two acromegalic patients: a double-blind study with long-term follow-up. Pain 1993; 53(2):223–227.

64. Pascual J, Freijanes J, Berciano J, Pesquera C. Analgesic effect of octreotide in headache associated with acromegaly is not mediated by opioid mechanisms. Case report. Pain 1991; 47(3):341–344.

65. Popovic V, Paunovic VR, Micic D, Nesovic M, Kendereski A, Djordjevic P, Manojlovic D, Micic J. The analgesic effect and development of dependency to somatostatin analogue (octreotide) in headache associated with acromegaly. Horm Metab Res 1988; 20(4):250–251.

66. Williams G, Ball JA, Lawson RA, Joplin GF, Bloom SR, Maskill MR. Analgesic effect of somatostatin analogue (octreotide) in headache associated with pituitary tumours. Br Med J (Clin Res Ed) 1987; 295(6592):247–248.

67. Colao A, Cannavo S, Marzullo P, Pivonello R, Squadrito S, Vallone G, Almoto B, Bichisao E, Trimarchi F, Lombardi G. Twelve months of treatment with octreotide-LAR reduces joint thickness in acromegaly. Eur J Endocrinol 2003; 148(1):31–38.

68. Herrmann BL, Wessendorf TE, Ajaj W, Kahlke S, Teschler H, Mann K. Effects of octreotide on sleep apnoea and tongue volume (magnetic resonance imaging) in patients with acromegaly. Eur J Endocrinol 2004; 151(3):309–315.

69. Ip MS, Tan KC, Peh WC, Lam KS. Effect of Sandostatin LAR on sleep apnoea in acromegaly: correlation with computerized tomographic cephalometry and hormonal activity. Clin Endocrinol (Oxf) 2001; 55(4):477–483.

70. Chanson P, Timsit J, Benoit O, Augendre B, Moulonguet M, Guillausseau PG, Warnet A, Lubetzki J. Rapid improvement in sleep apnoea of acromegaly after short-term treatment with somatostatin analogue SMS 201-995. Lancet 1986; 1(8492):1270–1271.

71. Leibowitz G, Shapiro MS, Salameh M, Glaser B. Improvement of sleep apnoea due to acromegaly during short-term treatment with octreotide. J Intern Med 1994; 236(2):231–235.

72. Grunstein RR, Ho KK, Sullivan CE. Effect of octreotide, a somatostatin analog, on sleep apnea in patients with acromegaly. Ann Intern Med 1994; 121(7):478–483.

7

Growth Hormone Receptor Antagonist

THE DEVELOPMENT OF PEGVISOMANT

The growth hormone receptor (GHR) antagonist pegvisomant is the newest modality for the treatment of acromegaly. The design and development of pegvisomant came about as a result of experiments into the structural–functional relationship between growth hormone (GH) and its receptor. It is now known that GH activates its receptor in a two-step process that involves receptor dimerization: First, a GH molecule binds to a GH receptor at what is called binding site 1; then the GH molecule binds to a second GH receptor via a second site, binding site 2. Thereafter, signaling is induced and the receptor dimer complex is internalized.

The GH molecule is 191 amino acids in length and is organized in a series of four α-helices that are connected by nonhelical regions (1). It was noted that the third α-helix was amphipathic in structure, with hydrophilic and hydrophobic residues grouped together, although the amphipathic structure was imperfect at three amino acids in the bovine GH molecule. Kopchick's group (2) undertook a series of mutagenesis experiments to "correct" the third helix and give it a perfect amphipathic structure, supposing that this would augment GH receptor activation. In direct contrast, this altered GH molecule led to dwarfism in transgenic mice, and although GH levels were high in these animals, IGF-I levels were suppressed. It was found subsequently that when a glycine residue at position 119 (Gly-119) in the third α-helix was replaced by a larger amino acid, this interfered with GH–GH receptor binding at binding site 2. Thus, GH receptor dimerization was abrogated by this single amino acid change, and subsequent intracellular activation cascades and downstream effects, such as IGF-I secretion, were prevented. It was shown subsequently that similar replacement of the analogous glycine in human GH at position 120 produced the same effect.

Given the profound inhibition of GH action by this mutated GH molecule, it was recognized that this could have therapeutic benefits. Subsequently, modifications were made to the altered GH molecule to augment its affinity for the GH receptor at binding site 1 to increase its pharmacologic antagonism of the GH receptor. Also, the half-life of the altered GH molecule was increased compared with that of native GH by adding a series of polyethylene glycol residues (Figs. 1 and 2). This growth hormone receptor antagonist–with increased affinity for the GH receptor at binding site 1–altered binding site 2 structure that prevents GH receptor dimerization, and a long half-life due to pegylation—is known as pegvisomant (3). Subsequent studies have shown that pegylation reduces the clearance of pegvisomant, presumably via decreased renal excretion, while it also reduces interactions with the circulating GH binding protein (4). These beneficial pharmacological effects of pegylation come at a cost of decreased GH receptor affinity compared with the non-pegylated GH receptor antagonist molecule (4). Pegvisomant appears

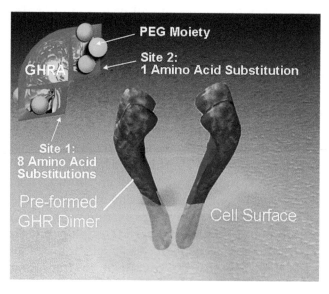

Figure 1
Alterations to the binding sites of pegvisomant to the growth hormone receptor (GHR). PEG, polyethylene glycol.

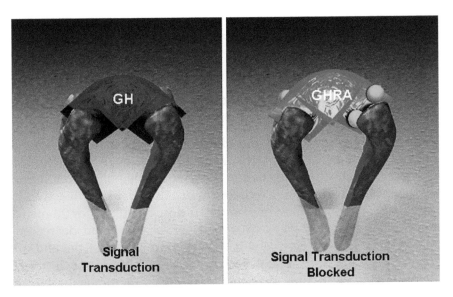

Figure 2
Dimerization of the growth hormone receptor by GH leads to signal transduction
(*left*), while the binding site mutations allow pegvisomant to bind with high
affinity to binding site 1, but prevent proper dimerization via alteration of
binding site 2.

to bind specifically to the GH receptor, and has no cross-reactivity with
prolactin receptors in vitro (5). After pegvisomant binds to the GH receptor dimer and blocks signal transduction, the pegvisomant–GH receptor
complex is cleared from the membrane surface by internalization (6).

Data from a phase I study of pegvisomant in healthy male volunteers
were supportive of the potential for using pegvisomant to reduce IGF-I
hypersecretion in acromegaly. Thorner et al. (7) reported that a single subcutaneous injection of 1.0 mg/kg pegvisomant reduced IGF-I measured 7
days later by approximately 50%.

PEGVISOMANT IN THE TREATMENT
OF ACROMEGALY

Effects on the GH–IGF-I Axis

Pegvisomant has a range of actions on the activity of the GH–IGF-I axis in
humans. Acute administration of pegvisomant in healthy subjects and
long-term administration in patients with acromegaly are associated with
dose-related suppression of serum IGF-I (7–9). From data in healthy
volunteers, the effect of pegvisomant appears to be to reduce serum free
IGF-I, with consequently increased GH concentrations possibly mediated
via an increased GHRH response (10). Pegvisomant also decreases the

elevated levels of total IGFBP-3, acid-labile subunit and thus the 150 kDa ternary complex-associated IGFBP-3 seen in patients with active acromegaly (11).

Control of Hormonal Hypersecretion and Signs and Symptoms

Two large studies examining the effects of pegvisomant on signs and symptoms and hormonal control in acromegaly have been published (8,9). Trainer et al. (9) performed a 12-week, double-blind, randomized, placebo-controlled study of pegvisomant in 112 patients with active acromegaly. Pegvisomant was administered at doses of 10, 15, or 20 mg/day, and at the end of the 12-week treatment period, IGF-I had decreased by 27%, 50%, and 63%, respectively. IGF-I was normalized at the end of the study in 54%, 81%, and 89% of patients receiving 10, 15, or 20 mg/day of pegvisomant. Both ring size and a composite acromegaly symptom score consisting of the severities of soft tissue swelling, arthralgia, headache, perspiration, and fatigue decreased significantly in each pegvisomant-treated group compared with placebo (9).

The long-term safety and efficacy profile of pegvisomant in acromegaly was demonstrated in a study of 160 patients who were treated for up to 18 months (8). The mean age of the group was 46 years and the cohort consisted of 59% men and 41% women. The mean duration of disease before enrolment into the study was 8 years. The majority of patients had received previous therapy: 84% had undergone surgery, 73% had received somatostatin analogs, 59% had undergone radiotherapy, and 48% had received a dopamine agonist. After a washout period following withdrawal of somatostatin analogs (2 weeks) or dopamine agonists (5 weeks), patients who had an age-adjusted IGF-I 30% above the upper limit of normal were enrolled to receive pegvisomant starting at 10 mg/day, which was titrated up or down by 5 mg/day every 2–8 weeks until an age-adjusted normal IGF-I was achieved. Patients were divided into three cohorts for data analysis based on results obtained after 6 ($n = 131$), 12 ($n = 90$), or 18 ($n = 39$) months of pegvisomant therapy. The mean treatment duration for patients receiving pegvisomant was 425 days, and a total of 186 patient-years of pegvisomant were recorded in the study. The mean doses in the three cohorts were 14.7 mg/day (6 months), 18.0 mg/day (12 months), and 19.6 mg/day (18 months). In 97% (87/90) of patients treated for $\geq$12 months, a normal age-adjusted IGF-I concentration was achieved during the study (Fig. 3). GH levels, as measured by a special assay that was saturated for the non-pegylated parent molecule of pegvisomant, rose concomitantly as IGF-I decreased. This rise in GH normalized within 30 days of pegvisomant withdrawal. One important caveat for pegvisomant treatment of acromegaly is the avoidance of functional GH deficiency due to potent suppression of IGF-I secretion.

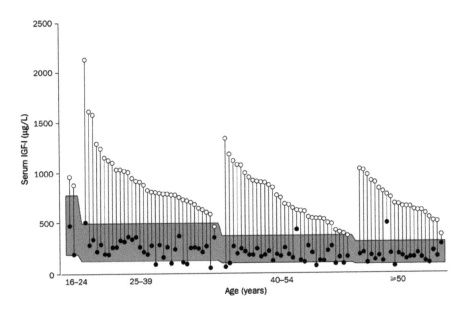

Figure 3

Baseline (open circles) and nadir (filled circles) levels of IGF-I from 90 individual patients with acromegaly treated daily for 12 months or more with pegvisomant. The green shaded region represents the normal, age-adjusted range of IGF-I.
Source: Reprinted with permission from Elsevier (*The Lancet*, 2001; 358(9295):1754–1759).

During treatment with pegvisomant for more than 1 year, 11 of 90 patients experienced IGF-I levels below the age-adjusted lower limit of normal (8). This can be readily avoided by close follow-up of IGF-I levels and dose titration to the median of the normal range adjusted for the age and sex of the patient.

Patients who are resistant to surgery and/or radiotherapy plus medical therapy and have persistent disease activity can also benefit from pegvisomant. A group of seven such patients with multimodal treatment-resistant acromegaly experienced normalization of IGF-I and improvements in signs and symptoms during treatment with pegvisomant (15–40 mg/day) for up to 2 years (12).

Carbohydrate Metabolism

Glucose intolerance and diabetes due to insulin resistance occur frequently in acromegaly (13,14), while normalization of GH/IGF-I hypersecretion with surgery or radiotherapy is associated with improved carbohydrate metabolism (15–17). In contrast, somatostatin analog treatment of acromegaly can worsen glycemic control in some patients (18). The difference between pegvisomant and somatostatin analogs in this regard is due in part to the inhibitory effects of somatostatin analogs on gastrointestinal hormones, including glucagon and insulin. Short-term studies in healthy volunteers have confirmed this by comparing the effects of pegvisomant (20 mg/day) and octreotide (50 μg every 8 hr for 7 days) on carbohydrate metabolism and gastrointestinal hormones. Pegvisomant did not impact post-OGTT glucose tolerance or post-test-meal gut hormone release, while octreotide impaired glucose tolerance and inhibited insulin, cholecystokinin, gastrin, insulin, and pancreatic polypeptide secretion (19).

In a group of seven acromegalic patients, Drake et al. (20) demonstrated that fasting glucose fell when medication was switched from the somatostatin analog octreotide to pegvisomant. Furthermore, four patients on octreotide who had impaired fasting glucose or glucose levels indicative of diabetes mellitus experienced normalization of glucose concentrations on pegvisomant. The improvements seen in the study were due largely to improved peripheral insulin sensitivity during pegvisomant therapy and occurred at similar levels of IGF-I control with both treatments. These results were borne out by long-term data in 160 patients treated for up to 18 months (8). Fasting serum glucose concentrations fell significantly from baseline with pegvisomant after 6, 12, and 18 months of therapy. This improvement in glycemic control came in parallel with a significant decrease in serum insulin concentrations at the same timepoints, indicating improved insulin sensitivity in this large group.

Bone Markers

Acromegaly is characterized by the occurrence of bone and joint pathology (21,22). In uncontrolled disease, bone turnover is increased (23–26) and patients exhibit decreased biomechanical competence and density of trabecular bone (27). Two studies have been performed with pegvisomant in acromegaly to examine the effects of IGF-I normalization on bone turnover. Fairfield et al. measured markers of bone turnover [bone formation: serum procollagen I carboxy-terminal propeptide (PICP), osteocalcin; bone resorption: N-telopeptide (NTx)] in 27 patients with active acromegaly who received placebo or 10–20 mg of pegvisomant for 3 months. Pegvisomant treatment was associated with a decrease in IGF-I, which was accompanied by a significant fall in measures of both bone formation and resorption compared with baseline (28). In a second study involving 16 patients with active acromegaly and 32 matched controls, those with acromegaly had significantly elevated levels of procollagen III amino-terminal propeptide (PIIINP), osteocalcin, and C-telopeptide (CTx) at baseline compared with controls. Normalization of IGF-I levels with pegvisomant was associated with decreased PIIINP, osteocalcin, CTx, NTx, and 1,25-dihydroxy-vitamin D. Parathyroid hormone rose and calcium clearance fell significantly from baseline in the acromegalic group. Pegvisomant-related changes brought the pattern of bone and connective tissue turnover in the acromegalic group in line with that seen in the normal control population (29).

Body Composition

Leptin is an important regulator of energy balance that is correlated with body fat mass and is increased in patients with GH deficiency (who have increased fat mass) and decreased in those with acromegaly (who have reduced fat mass) (30–32). The relationship between leptin and the GH–IGF-I axis appears to be indirect and mediated through alterations in adipose content and body composition (30); the role of carbohydrate metabolism in leptin regulation is uncertain (33,34). Both normal and acromegalic females have higher leptin levels than males, reflecting recognized differences in lean and fat body mass (35). Control of GH–IGF-I axis hypersecretion in acromegaly is associated with a rise in leptin concentrations in line with changes in body mass index (36). Parkinson et al. (37) studied the effect of pegvisomant treatment on serum leptin levels in 16 patients with active acromegaly. As expected, females had higher levels than males at baseline, and the levels correlated with body mass index. After IGF-I normalization following a mean of 7 months of pegvisomant therapy at a median dose of 20 mg/day, serum leptin rose significantly. The percentage rise in leptin was greater in male acromegalic patients than in females. As there was no change in bound leptin or serum leptin receptors, it was concluded that IGF-I normalization by pegvisomant in acromegaly increases free leptin concentrations.

Cortisol Metabolism

GH has an inhibitory effect on one isoform of 11-β-hydroxysteroid dehydrogenase that is responsible for interconverting cortisone and cortisol. Trainer et al. (38) studied the effect of GH antagonism on urinary measures of 11-β-hydroxysteroid dehydrogenase activity in seven patients with active acromegaly over a mean period of 46 weeks of treatment. A rise in the urinary measures occurred concomitant with a significant decrease/normalization of IGF-I secretion. The authors suggested that these data could have implications for the calculation of glucocorticoid replacement dosages in patients with or without active acromegaly.

ADVERSE EVENTS

Tumor Size

Pegvisomant treatment of acromegaly with regular MRI follow-up over a period of up to 18 months was not associated with an overall change in tumor size from baseline (8). At entry, mean tumor volume in 160 patients was 2.39 ± 3.45 cm^3. At 6, 12, and 18 months, tumor volume on MRI was 2.14 ± 2.47 (131 patients), 2.44 ± 2.70 (90 patients), and 2.49 ± 2.58 cm^3 (39 patients). No association was seen between pegvisomant treatment duration and tumor volume change. When individual patients were considered, two cases of tumor growth were noted to have occurred during the study. In both cases, patients had large, globular, aggressive tumors that had proven resistant to pituitary surgery. Neither patient had received previous radiotherapy, and there was optical chiasmal impingement in both cases. One patient received pegvisomant on and off (due to an interruption in supply for 6 months) over a 15-month period before undergoing radiotherapy due to tumor expansion. In the other case, the 34-year-old male patient had a large tumor with optic chiasmal impingement 6 months after transsphenoidal surgery (39). He demonstrated a partial response to octreotide therapy and was also relatively resistant to pegvisomant at a dose of 40 mg/day, as he eventually demonstrated escape of IGF-I suppression. When this occurred, visual symptoms appeared and he was treated successfully with a combination of octreotide and pegvisomant. Pegvisomant withdrawal was associated with a return of symptoms, which were resistant to maximal doses of octreotide LAR, and surgical intervention was eventually required.

All patients with GH-secreting pituitary adenomas, including those receiving pegvisomant, should be monitored regularly for signs and symptoms of tumor growth. MRI scans should be performed on a regular basis in patients with significant residual tumor mass to identify tumor growth at an early stage.

Liver Function Tests

During 12 weeks of treatment of 160 acromegalic patients with pegvisomant, two cases (0.8%) of raised liver enzyme levels were noted (9). In these cases, hepatic aminotransferase levels were raised above ten times the upper limit of normal without increases in bilirubin concentration. Pegvisomant was withdrawn in both cases, and liver enzymes returned to normal. In one patient, a rechallenge with pegvisomant was associated with a repeated elevation in transaminase concentrations, while in the second case a liver biopsy showed chronic hepatitis of unknown origin. Patients should have liver enzymes measured at baseline before starting pegvisomant and every month thereafter for the first 6 months of therapy, every 3 months for the next 6 months, and then every 6 months for the next year. Increases in liver enzymes of 3–5 times the upper limit of normal without symptoms of hepatic damage or raised bilirubin should be followed weekly, and the patient should undergo a comprehensive workup. Any increase in bilirubin or signs/symptoms of hepatic damage necessitates withdrawal of pegvisomant and a thorough re-evaluation of liver function.

Antibodies

During long-term treatment, approximately 17% of patients developed antibodies to pegvisomant, mainly in low titers; antibodies to GH were also seen in the majority of these patients (8). Tachyphylaxis or other effects of such antibodies have not been reported to date during pegvisomant therapy.

PEGVISOMANT: INDICATIONS FOR TREATMENT

Surgery is the treatment of choice for patients with acromegaly. For cases not controlled by surgery, the options consist of pharmacotherapy, radiotherapy, or second surgery. Pharmacotherapy should be prescribed based on the characteristics of each individual patient and in line with the labeling guidelines of the territory. As pegvisomant is a relatively new therapy, its place in the treatment algorithm is still evolving (40). At present, the recommendations for when to use pegvisomant differ slightly in various jurisdictions, such as the United States and the European Union. In the United States, pegvisomant is currently indicated "for the treatment of acromegaly in patients who have an inadequate response to surgery and/or radiotherapy and/or medical therapies or for whom these therapies are not appropriate. The goal of treatment is to normalize serum IGF-I levels." In the European Union, the current recommendations are that pegvisomant is for the "treatment of patients with acromegaly who have had an inadequate response to surgery and/or radiotherapy and in whom appropriate medical treatment with somatostatin analogs did not normalize IGF-I concentrations or was not tolerated." After surgery and/or medical therapy, the European Union authorities favor a trial of somatostatin analogs (i.e., adjuvant therapy) first before using pegvisomant, while the authorities in the United States permit the use of pegvisomant as primary or adjuvant therapy. Pegvisomant is administered once daily by subcutaneous injection, beginning with a single loading dose of 40mg under medical supervision (In the EU, the loading dose is 80mg). The starting dose of pegvisomant is 10mg once daily and this should be titrated in 5mg increments (to a maximum dose of 30mg per day) every 4–6 weeks to achieve a normal age- and sex-matched IGF-I level.

REFERENCES

1. de Vos AM, Ultsch M, Kossiakoff AA. Human growth hormone and extracellular domain of its receptor: crystal structure of the complex. Science 1992; 255(5042):306–312.
2. Kopchick JJ. Discovery and development of a new class of drugs: GH antagonists. J Endocrinol Invest 2003; 26(suppl 10):16–26.
3. USAN Council. List No.428. New names. Pegvisomant. Clin Pharmacol Ther 2000; 68(1):106.
4. Ross RJ, Leung KC, Maamra M, Bennett W, Doyle N, Waters MJ, Ho KK. Binding and functional studies with the growth hormone receptor antagonist,

B2036-PEG (pegvisomant), reveal effects of pegylation and evidence that it binds to a receptor dimer. J Clin Endocrinol Metab 2001; 86(4):1716–1723.

5. Goffin V, Bernichtein S, Carriere O, Bennett WF, Kopchick JJ, Kelly PA. The human growth hormone antagonist B2036 does not interact with the prolactin receptor. Endocrinology 1999; 140(8):3853–3856.

6. Maamra M, Kopchick JJ, Strasburger CJ, Ross RJ. Pegvisomant, a growth hormone-specific antagonist, undergoes cellular internalization. J Clin Endocrinol Metab 2004; 89(9):4532–4537.

7. Thorner MO, Strasburger CJ, Wu Z, Straume M, Bidlingmaier M, Pezzoli SS, Zib K, Scarlett JC, Bennett WF. Growth hormone (GH) receptor blockade with a PEG-modified GH (B2036-PEG) lowers serum insulin-like growth factor-I but does not acutely stimulate serum GH. J Clin Endocrinol Metab 1999; 84(6):2098–2103.

8. van der Lely AJ, Hutson RK, Trainer PJ, Besser GM, Barkan AL, Katznelson L, Klibanski A, Herman-Bonert V, Melmed S, Vance ML, Freda PU, Stewart PM, Friend KE, Clemmons DR, Johannsson G, Stavrou S, Cook DM, Phillips LS, Strasburger CJ, Hackett S, Zib KA, Davis RJ, Scarlett JA, Thorner MO. Long-term treatment of acromegaly with pegvisomant, a growth hormone receptor antagonist. Lancet 2001; 358(9295):1754–1759.

9. Trainer PJ, Drake WM, Katznelson L, Freda PU, Herman-Bonert V, van der Lely AJ, Dimaraki EV, Stewart PM, Friend KE, Vance ML, Besser GM, Scarlett JA, Thorner MO, Parkinson C, Klibanski A, Powell JS, Barkan AL, Sheppard MC, Malsonado M, Rose DR, Clemmons DR, Johannsson G, Bengtsson BA, Stavrou S, Kleinberg DL, Cook DM, Phillips LS, Bidlingmaier M, Strasburger CJ, Hackett S, Zib K, Bennett WF, Davis RJ. Treatment of acromegaly with the growth hormone-receptor antagonist pegvisomant. N Engl J Med 2000; 342(16):1171–1177.

10. Muller AF, Janssen JA, Lamberts SW, Bidlingmaier M, Strasburger CJ, Hofland L, van der Lely AJ. Effects of fasting and pegvisomant on the GH-releasing hormone and GH-releasing peptide-6 stimulated growth hormone secretion. Clin Endocrinol (Oxf) 2001; 55(4):461–467.

11. Parkinson C, Flyvbjerg A, Trainer PJ. High levels of 150-kDa insulin-like growth factor binding protein three ternary complex in patients with acromegaly and the effect of pegvisomant-induced serum IGF-I normalization. Growth Horm IGF Res 2004; 14(1):59–65.

12. Drake WM, Parkinson C, Akker SA, Monson JP, Besser GM, Trainer PJ. Successful treatment of resistant acromegaly with a growth hormone receptor antagonist. Eur J Endocrinol 2001; 145(4):451–456.

13. Kasayama S, Otsuki M, Takagi M, Saito H, Sumitani S, Kouhara H, Koga M, Saitoh Y, Ohnishi T, Arita N. Impaired beta-cell function in the presence of reduced insulin sensitivity determines glucose tolerance status in acromegalic patients. Clin Endocrinol (Oxf) 2000; 52(5):549–555.

14. Colao A, Ferone D, Marzullo P, Lombardi G. Systemic complications of acromegaly: epidemiology, pathogenesis, and management. Endocr Rev 2004; 25(1):102–152.

15. Jaffrain-Rea ML, Minniti G, Moroni C, Esposito V, Ferretti E, Santoro A, Infusino T, Tamburrano G, Cantore G, Cassone R. Impact of successful transsphenoidal surgery on cardiovascular risk factors in acromegaly. Eur J Endocrinol 2003; 148(2):193–201.

16. Jaffrain-Rea ML, Moroni C, Baldelli R, Battista C, Maffei P, Terzolo M, Correra M, Ghiggi MR, Ferretti E, Angeli A, Sicolo N, Trischitta V, Liuzzi A, Cassone R, Tamburrano G. Relationship between blood pressure and glucose tolerance in acromegaly. Clin Endocrinol (Oxf) 2001; 54(2):189–195.

17. Barrande G, Pittino-Lungo M, Coste J, Ponvert D, Bertagna X, Luton JP, Bertherat J. Hormonal and metabolic effects of radiotherapy in acromegaly: long-term results in 128 patients followed in a single center. J Clin Endocrinol Metab 2000; 85(10):3779–3785.

18. Koop BL, Harris AG, Ezzat S. Effect of octreotide on glucose tolerance in acromegaly. Eur J Endocrinol 1994; 130(6):581–586.

19. Parkinson C, Drake WM, Roberts ME, Meeran K, Besser GM, Trainer PJ. A comparison of the effects of pegvisomant and octreotide on glucose, insulin, gastrin, cholecystokinin, and pancreatic polypeptide responses to oral glucose and a standard mixed meal. J Clin Endocrinol Metab 2002; 87(4):1797–1804.

20. Drake WM, Rowles SV, Roberts ME, Fode FK, Besser GM, Monson JP, Trainer PJ. Insulin sensitivity and glucose tolerance improve in patients with acromegaly converted from depot octreotide to pegvisomant. Eur J Endocrinol 2003; 149(6):521–527.

21. Nabarro JD. Acromegaly. Clin Endocrinol (Oxf) 1987; 26(4):481–512.

22. Ezzat S, Forster MJ, Berchtold P, Redelmeier DA, Boerlin V, Harris AG. Acromegaly. Clinical and biochemical features in 500 patients. Medicine (Baltimore) 1994; 73(5):233–240.

23. Marazuela M, Astigarraga B, Tabuenca MJ, Estrada J, Marin F, Lucas T. Serum bone Gla protein as a marker of bone turnover in acromegaly. Calcif Tissue Int 1993; 52(6):419–421.

24. Kotzmann H, Bernecker P, Hubsch P, Pietschmann P, Woloszczuk W, Svoboda T, Geyer G, Luger A. Bone mineral density and parameters of bone metabolism in patients with acromegaly. J Bone Miner Res 1993; 8(4): 459–465.

25. Terzolo M, Piovesan A, Osella G, Pia A, Reimondo G, Pozzi C, Raucci C, Torta M, Paccotti P, Angeli A. Serum levels of bone Gla protein (osteocalcin, BGP) and carboxyterminal propeptide of type I procollagen (PICP) in acromegaly: effects of long-term octreotide treatment. Calcif Tissue Int 1993; 52(3):188–191.

26. Lieberman SA, Bjorkengren AG, Hoffman AR. Rheumatologic and skeletal changes in acromegaly. Endocrinol Metab Clin North Am 1992; 21(3): 615–631.

27. Ueland T, Ebbesen EN, Thomsen JS, Mosekilde L, Brixen K, Flyvbjerg A, Bollerslev J. Decreased trabecular bone biomechanical competence, apparent

density, IGF-II and IGFBP-5 content in acromegaly. Eur J Clin Invest 2002; 32(2):122–128.

28. Fairfield WP, Sesmilo G, Katznelson L, Pulaski K, Freda PU, Stavrou S, Kleinberg D, Klibanski A. Effects of a growth hormone receptor antagonist on bone markers in acromegaly. Clin Endocrinol (Oxf) 2002; 57(3):385–390.

29. Parkinson C, Kassem M, Heickendorff L, Flyvbjerg A, Trainer PJ. Pegvisomant-induced serum insulin-like growth factor-I normalization in patients with acromegaly returns elevated markers of bone turnover to normal. J Clin Endocrinol Metab 2003; 88(12):5650–5655.

30. Bolanowski M, Milewicz A, Bidzinska B, Jedrzejuk D, Daroszewski J, Mikulski E. Serum leptin levels in acromegaly—a significant role for adipose tissue and fasting insulin/glucose ratio. Med Sci Monit 2002; 8(10):CR685–CR689.

31. Damjanovic SS, Petakov MS, Raicevic S, Micic D, Marinkovic J, Dieguez C, Casanueva FF, Popovic V. Serum leptin levels in patients with acromegaly before and after correction of hypersomatotropism by trans–sphenoidal surgery. J Clin Endocrinol Metab 2000; 85(1):147–154.

32. Miyakawa M, Tsushima T, Murakami H, Isozaki O, Demura H, Tanaka T. Effect of growth hormone (GH) on serum concentrations of leptin: study in patients with acromegaly and GH deficiency. J Clin Endocrinol Metab 1998; 83(10):3476–3479.

33. Silha JV, Krsek M, Hana V, Marek J, Jezkova J, Weiss V, Murphy LJ. Perturbations in adiponectin, leptin and resistin levels in acromegaly: lack of correlation with insulin resistance. Clin Endocrinol (Oxf) 2003; 58(6):736–742.

34. Adan L, Trivin C, Sainte–Rose C, Zucker JM, Hartmann O, Brauner R. GH deficiency caused by cranial irradiation during childhood: factors and markers in young adults. J Clin Endocrinol Metab 2001; 86(11):5245–5251.

35. Jorgensen JO, Vahl N, Dall R, Christiansen JS. Resting metabolic rate in healthy adults: relation to growth hormone status and leptin levels. Metabolism 1998; 47(9):1134–1139.

36. Tan KC, Tso AW, Lam KS. Effect of Sandostatin LAR on serum leptin levels in patients with acromegaly. Clin Endocrinol (Oxf) 2001; 54(1):31–35.

37. Parkinson C, Whatmore AJ, Yates AP, Drake WM, Brabant G, Clayton PE, Trainer PJ. The effect of pegvisomant-induced serum IGF-I normalization on serum leptin levels in patients with acromegaly. Clin Endocrinol (Oxf) 2003; 59(2):168–174.

38. Trainer PJ, Drake WM, Perry LA, Taylor NF, Besser GM, Monson JP. Modulation of cortisol metabolism by the growth hormone receptor antagonist pegvisomant in patients with acromegaly. J Clin Endocrinol Metab 2001; 86(7):2989–2992.

39. van der Lely AJ, Muller A, Janssen JA, Davis RJ, Zib KA, Scarlett JA, Lamberts SW. Control of tumor size and disease activity during cotreatment with octreotide and the growth hormone receptor antagonist pegvisomant in an acromegalic patient. J Clin Endocrinol Metab 2001; 86(2):478–481.

40. Clemmons DR, Chihara K, Freda PU, Ho KK, Klibanski A, Melmed S, Shalet SM, Strasburger CJ, Trainer PJ, Thorner MO. Optimizing control of acromegaly: integrating a growth hormone receptor antagonist into the treatment algorithm. J Clin Endocrinol Metab 2003; 88(10):4759–4767.

8

Dopamine Agonists

BACKGROUND

Dopamine acts to stimulate growth hormone (GH) release from the pituitary in normal individuals. However, in acromegaly, it has the opposite effect and inhibits GH secretion. While the explanation of this phenomenon is unclear, the inhibitory effect of dopamine on GH secretion has been used therapeutically to treat acromegaly for about 30 years (1–4). In approximately 30% of cases of acromegaly, the tumor is plurihormonal in nature and can secrete prolactin in addition to GH (5,6). Thus, acromegalic patients who have elevated prolactin levels represent the target population for dopamine agonist therapy.

CLINICAL STUDIES

The first dopamine agonist to be used to treat acromegaly in widespread clinical practice was the orally available ergot alkaloid bromocriptine (1–4). Since the early 1970s, well over one thousand patients with acromegaly have received bromocriptine in the clinical trial setting. In 1992, Jaffe and Barkan (7) undertook an extensive review of studies of bromocriptine in acromegaly published during the previous two decades. The efficacy of bromocriptine varies according to the criteria used to interpret what constitutes control of acromegaly. Of 549 patients in 31 studies in which the cut-off for GH control was $<10\,\mu g/L$, the cure rate was approximately 50% (7). When the threshold for cure was lowered to a GH level $<5\,\mu g/L$, the cure rate dropped to about 20%. Insulin-like growth factor-I (IGF-I) normalization occurred in only 10% of patients treated. Clinical response to bromocriptine was adequate overall, with reductions in symptoms and signs of acromegaly, but little evidence of tumor shrinkage.

Since the introduction of bromocriptine, a group of more potent ergot and non-ergot dopamine agonists have been developed for acromegaly, including lisuride (8), pergolide (9), and quinagolide (10,11), and all have proven effective for long-term control, although control rates are a function of the definition used. Indeed, many of these studies expressed efficacy only in terms of percentage decreases in GH secretion (e.g., a 50% decrease) during treatment (8,9,12,13).

Chief among the newer dopamine agonists is cabergoline, which is a long-acting, synthetic ergot derivative that is relatively selective for the dopamine D_2 receptor as compared with bromocriptine. In an early study in 1988, Ferrari (14) studied the effects of single doses of 0.3 and 0.6 mg of cabergoline on GH and prolactin secretion in dopamine agonist responsive acromegalic patients. The effects of cabergoline on prolactin secretion were rapid and endured for up to 7 days post-dose. GH decreased significantly (42% after 1 day) for up to 3 days after 0.6 mg of cabergoline. During once-weekly therapy, 50% of patients (3 of 6) achieved a normalized IGF-I level, and improvements in GH and IGF-I control were seen in the remaining 50% of patients following cabergoline dose increases (14). Larger long-term studies in acromegaly have also been performed using cabergoline. In the largest of these, 64 patients with active acromegaly received cabergoline at 1.0 mg/week, which was titrated upward to a maximum of 3.5–7.0 mg/week or until IGF-I was normalized or unacceptable adverse events occurred (15). IGF-I levels decreased to $\leq 450\,\mu g/L$ in 67% of patients, and to $<300\,\mu g/L$ in 39% of the group overall. Suppression of IGF-I was determined partially by the pretreatment IGF-I, as patients with a pretreatment IGF-I $<750\,\mu g/L$ had a higher rate of response to cabergoline than those with an IGF-I $>750\,\mu g/L$.

Cozzi et al. (16) reported the results of an open label study in 18 patients with acromegaly who received cabergoline at doses equivalent to 1–3.5 mg/week. In comparison with previous bromocriptine, cabergoline demonstrated greater efficacy in terms of hormonal control in this series. During treatment, basal GH decreased significantly from 6.6 to $3.5\,\mu g/L$, while IGF-I decreased from 720 to $375\,\mu g/L$. Normal age-adjusted IGF-I values were attained in 27% of the series.

Two studies have examined the possibility of combining cabergoline therapy with a somatostatin analog to improve GH/IGF-I control (17,18). Marzullo et al.(18). studied the effect of lanreotide treatment for a 6-month period with or without cabergoline in ten patients with acromegaly who were relatively resistant to octreotide or octreotide/quinagolide. After 3 months of lanreotide/cabergoline combination therapy, GH was suppressed to $< 2.5\,\mu g/L$ in four patients and IGF-I was normalized in five. The additive effects of cabergoline and lanreotide on GH and IGF-I secretion were greater than either therapy alone. In a subgroup of seven patients, no change in tumor size was seen on MRI (18).

In another study, Cozzi et al. (17) examined the effects on biochemical control of the addition of cabergoline to pre-existing octreotide therapy. A total of 19 acromegalic patients with active disease, who were resistant to octreotide LAR or lanreotide SR therapy, were tested. Combined treatment lowered GH to $< 2.5\,\mu g/L$ in 21% of cases and normalized IGF-I for age in eight patients (42%).

The rates and extent of tumor shrinkage with dopamine agonists in acromegaly have not been studied extensively, although it is clear that the sizable tumor reduction seen in dopamine agonist-treated prolactinomas is not broadly achievable in acromegaly. Clinical studies indicate that GH or GH/prolactin-secreting pituitary adenomas occasionally shrink with the various available dopamine agonists, and there are no data to suggest that any one dopamine agonist is more likely than the others to produce tumor shrinkage in acromegaly. For instance, Colao et al. reported tumor shrinkage of $> 30\%$ in 3 of 34 patients (8.8%) with acromegaly treated with either bromocriptine (1/7), cabergoline (0/11), or quinagolide ($n = 2/16$) for 6–12 months (19). Only one of these three patients with tumor shrinkage exhibited hyperprolactinemia. Another study of cabergoline demonstrated no tumor shrinkage in a series of 14 acromegalic patients with active disease postoperatively, despite a significant decrease in GH levels and a temporary fall in IGF-I secretion (20). Interestingly, this study also reported the case of a separate patient with a large GH and prolactin co-secreting pituitary tumor that experienced progressive tumor shrinkage over a 4-year period of treatment with cabergoline alone. This patient also exhibited normalization of GH, IGF-I, and prolactin levels and disappearance of signs and symptoms of acromegaly and associated hypogonadism. Overall, clinically relevant tumor shrinkage can occur in a minority of acromegalic patients treated with dopamine agonists, and in individual cases this shrinkage can be sizable.

The use of dopamine agonist/somatostatin analog combinations, and their relative ability to induce hormonal suppression, has led to efforts to develop a bi-agonistic molecule. Such a chimeric somatostatin–dopamine agonist, BIM-23A387, has been studied in cell cultures of pituitary adenomas from acromegalic patients (21). This molecule has affinity for somatostatin receptor subtype 2 and the D_2 dopamine receptor. BIM-23A387 inhibited GH release from cultured pituitary tumor cells to an extent similar to that of either specific D_2 agonists or somatostatin receptor subtype 2-specific somatostatin analogs. In tumors that were poorly responsive to either dopamine agonist or somatostatin analogs alone,

BIM-23A387 produced dose-related suppression of GH. Further characterization of this and similar molecules is required in in vivo models to determine whether such chimeric molecules are promising for development as pharmacotherapeutics.

ADVERSE EVENTS

Adverse events attributable to dopamine agonists include nausea, vomiting, abdominal cramping, orthostatic hypotension, and dizziness. Older dopamine agonists such as bromocriptine exhibit greater adverse event profiles than newer agents. Some of these adverse events can be avoided by titrating up from lower doses, taking medication when going to bed, and having a snack before dosing.

REFERENCES

1. Sachdev Y, Gomez-Pan A, Tunbridge WM, Duns A, Weightman DR, Hall R, Goolamali SK. Bromocriptine therapy in acromegaly. Lancet 1975; 2(7946):1164–1168.

2. Summers VK, Hipkin LJ, Diver MH, Davis JC. Treatment of acromegaly with bromocryptine. J Clin Endocrinol Metab 1975; 40(5):904–906.

3. Thorner MO, Chait A, Aitken M, Benker G, Bloom SR, Mortimer CH, Sanders P, Mason AS, Besser GM. Bromocriptine treatment of acromegaly. Br Med J 1975; 1(5953):299–303.

4. Liuzzi A, Chiodini PG, Botalla L, Cremascoli G, Muller EE, Silvestrini F. Decreased plasma growth hormone (GH) levels in acromegalics following CB 154(2-Br-alpha ergocryptine) administration. J Clin Endocrinol Metab 1974; 38(5):910–912.

5. Lloyd RV, Cano M, Chandler WF, Barkan AL, Horvath E, Kovacs K. Human growth hormone and prolactin secreting pituitary adenomas analyzed by in situ hybridization. Am J Pathol 1989; 134(3):605–613.

6. Lloyd RV, Anagnostou D, Cano M, Barkan AL, Chandler WF. Analysis of mammosomatotropic cells in normal and neoplastic human pituitary tissues by the reverse hemolytic plaque assay and immunocytochemistry. J Clin Endocrinol Metab 1988; 66(6):1103–1110.

7. Jaffe CA, Barkan AL. Treatment of acromegaly with dopamine agonists. Endocrinol Metab Clin North Am 1992; 21(3):713–735.

8. Liuzzi A, Chiodini PG, Oppizzi G, Botalla L, Verde G, De Stefano L, Colussi G, Graf KJ, Horowski R. Lisuride hydrogen maleate: evidence for a long lasting dopaminergic activity in humans. J Clin Endocrinol Metab 1978; 46(2):196–202.

9. Kendall–Taylor P, Upstill–Goddard G, Cook D. Longterm pergolide treatment of acromegaly. Clin Endocrinol (Oxf) 1983; 19(6):711–719.

10. Ferone D, Pivonello R, Lastoria S, Faggiano A, Del Basso de Caro ML, Cappabianca P, Lombardi G, Colao A. In vivo and in vitro effects of octreotide, quinagolide and cabergoline in four hyperprolactinaemic acromegalics: correlation with somatostatin and dopamine D2 receptor scintigraphy. Clin Endocrinol (Oxf) 2001; 54(4):469–477.

11. Nickelsen T, Jungmann E, Althoff P, Schumm–Draeger PM, Usadel KH. Treatment of macroprolactinoma with the new potent non-ergot D2-dopamine agonist quinagolide and effects on prolactin levels, pituitary function, an the renin-aldosterone system. Results of a clinical long–term study. Arzneimittelforschung 1993; 43(4):421–425.

12. Oppizzi G, Liuzzi A, Chiodini P, Dallabonzana D, Spelta B, Silvestrini F, Borghi G, Tonon C. Dopaminergic treatment of acromegaly: different effects on hormone secretion and tumor size. J Clin Endocrinol Metab 1984; 58(6):988–992.

13. Kleinberg DL, Boyd AE III, Wardlaw S, Frantz AG, George A, Bryan N, Hilal S, Greising J, Hamilton D, Seltzer T, Sommers CJ. Pergolide for the treatment of pituitary tumors secreting prolactin or growth hormone. N Engl J Med 1983; 309(12):704–709.

14. Ferrari C, Paracchi A, Romano C, Gerevini G, Boghen M, Barreca A, Fortini P, Dubini A. Long-lasting lowering of serum growth hormone and prolactin levels by single and repetitive cabergoline administration in dopamine-responsive acromegalic patients. Clin Endocrinol (Oxf) 1988; 29(5):467–476.

15. Abs R, Verhelst J, Maiter D, Van Acker K, Nobels F, Coolens JL, Mahler C, Beckers A. Cabergoline in the treatment of acromegaly: a study in 64 patients. J Clin Endocrinol Metab 1998; 83(2):374–378.

16. Cozzi R, Attanasio R, Barausse M, Dallabonzana D, Orlandi P, Da Re N, Branca V, Oppizzi G, Gelli D. Cabergoline in acromegaly: a renewed role for dopamine agonist treatment? Eur J Endocrinol 1998; 139(5):516–521.

17. Cozzi R, Attanasio R, Lodrini S, Lasio G. Cabergoline addition to depot somatostatin analogues in resistant acromegalic patients: efficacy and lack of predictive value of prolactin status. Clin Endocrinol (Oxf) 2004; 61(2):209–215.

18. Marzullo P, Ferone D, Di Somma C, Pivonello R, Filippella M, Lombardi G, Colao A. Efficacy of combined treatment with lanreotide and cabergoline in selected therapy–resistant acromegalic patients. Pituitary 1999; 1(2):115–120.

19. Colao A, Ferone D, Marzullo P, Di Sarno A, Cerbone G, Sarnacchiaro F, Cirillo S, Merola B, Lombardi G. Effect of different dopaminergic agents in the treatment of acromegaly. J Clin Endocrinol Metab 1997; 82(2):518–523.

20. Freda PU, Reyes CM, Nuruzzaman AT, Sundeen RE, Khandji AG, Post KD. Cabergoline therapy of growth hormone and growth hormone/prolactin secreting pituitary tumors. Pituitary 2004; 7(1):21–30.

21. Saveanu A, Lavaque E, Gunz G, Barlier A, Kim S, Taylor JE, Culler MD, Enjalbert A, Jaquet P. Demonstration of enhanced potency of a chimeric somatostatin-dopamine molecule, BIM–23A387, in suppressing growth hormone and prolactin secretion from human pituitary somatotroph adenoma cells. J Clin Endocrinol Metab 2002; 87(12):5545–5552.

Radiotherapy

BACKGROUND

Radiotherapy for acromegaly has been used for nearly a century, either alone or as an adjuvant to neurosurgery (1). The methods used for external beam radiation of small targets that lie in close proximity to other vital structures have evolved greatly. It is now possible to deliver an effective dose of radiotherapy to a pituitary adenoma in one or more sessions, while minimizing radiation effects on the remaining pituitary, cranial nerves, and brain. This chapter provides a brief description of each of the modern methods used in radiotherapy, reviews the disease control afforded by each modality, and highlights adverse event profiles.

EFFICACY OF RADIOTHERAPY IN ACROMEGALY

Fractionated External Beam Radiotherapy

Conventional radiotherapy has been in use for many decades and utilizes equipment such as a linear accelerator to produce mega-electron volt beams. The tumor and surrounding structures, such as the remaining pituitary and the optic nerves, are mapped out accurately using MRI scans and the radiotherapy field is plotted. The patient is fitted with a specially designed plastic head mask and is immobilized, usually at an elevation of 30 degrees from the horizontal to decrease exposure of the optic nerves to radiation (1). The head is positioned precisely using fixed points on the patient's skull to permit absolute reproducibility during multiple sessions. Simulation is used to verify positioning before radiotherapy begins. Three beams, two lateral and one oblique anterior, are usually used. Currently doses of 1.8 Gy per day to a total of 45 Gy are recommended to reduce adverse events (2).

Eastman et al. (1) reviewed extensive data on the use of fractionated external beam radiotherapy in patients with acromegaly up to the beginning of the 1990s. As with other therapies discussed in this book, the efficacy of treatment in historical series can be misleading, as the cutoffs that were used to define normalization of GH and IGF-I were higher than those used today. In their own series of patients from the National Institutes of Health, Eastman et al. reported that growth hormone (GH) levels of <5 ng/mL were reached in 77% of patients at 15 years post-radiotherapy and in 88% of those followed for more than 15 years (1). Improvements in symptoms of acromegaly accompanied these decreases in GH secretion; however, the onset was slow. When modern criteria are applied to the control of acromegaly with radiotherapy, the results are less impressive in the short term. Using normal age-matched insulin-like growth factor-I (IGF-I) as the measure of control, Barkan and co-workers reported that only 35.5% of patients were controlled during follow-up of 4–15 years (3). A further study from Minniti et al reported that GH control (defined as a GH <1 μg/L post oral glucose tolerance test (OGTT) was achieved in 9%, 29%, 52% and 77% of acromegalic patients 2, 5, 10, and 15 years post external radiotherapy (4). IGF-I was controlled in 8%, 23%, 42%, and 61% of patients after 2, 5, 10 and 15 years of follow up.

The control of tumor growth with radiotherapy is good, with only 0.3% exhibiting continued growth in the Eastman et al. analysis. These data have been supported by Brada et al. (5), who showed that close to 90% of patients who received radiotherapy (with or without surgery) remained progression-free 20 years later.

Stereotactic Conformal Radiotherapy

This approach differs from conventional external beam radiotherapy in that it uses multiple fields (5–7 fields have been reported) in different planes to target radiation that conforms to the shape of the tumor contour (6,7). The patient undergoes immobilization and stereotactic localization of the tumor and surrounding structures, and the tumor is delineated using CT or MRI. A three-dimensional calculation of total tumor volume is made, and the radiotherapy dosing is planned using specialized computer software. Radiation is generated using a linear accelerator, and stereotactic conformal radiotherapy delivers fractionated radiation to a total dose of 45–50 Gy (6).

There is relatively little experience with this form of radiotherapy in patients with acromegaly. Jalali et al. (6) have reported preliminary data in six patients. One patient had normalization of post OGTT GH and IGF-I levels, four others had declining hormone levels, and one patient had an unresponsive GH secretion over 1–26 months of follow-up.

A recent study from Heidelberg, Germany reported experience with this method in 20 patients with acromegaly (8). After 26 months of follow-up, GH was normal (not defined) in 16 of 20 patients, although 5 required concomitant somatostatin analog therapy. IGF-I levels decreased in 9 of 20 patients, but normalization was not reported. Five patients with GH normalization had a reduction in tumor volume as measured by MRI.

Efficacy of Radiotherapy in Acromegaly

Radiosurgery is the name given to a selection of stereotactic approaches that deliver radiation to a tumor in one session. Three methods can be used for radiosurgery: gamma knife, a linear accelerator with a moving arc, and a cyclotron-based heavy beam generator in which the patient is moved. The gamma knife uses multiple gamma beams from a ^{60}Co source that are focused on a single discrete region of tumor. Multiple isocenters are generated using beams of different diameters in order to target irregularly sized tumors. Radiosurgical techniques target radiation quite precisely at the tumor; however, close proximity to a vital structure, such as the optic chiasma, limits their ability to deliver effective ablative doses.

Laws et al. (9) have recently published a comprehensive review and analysis of the literature on radiosurgery in the treatment of pituitary adenomas. They identified 25 studies concerning the use of radiosurgery in the treatment of 420 patients with acromegaly between 1993 and 2003. All but three of these studies used gamma knife; the others used a linear accelerator in very small numbers of patients (one to four). The mean radiosurgery dose was 15–34 Gy. Twelve different endocrinological cure or control definitions were used in 18 studies that reported such data. The overall 2-year endocrinological rate was between 20% and 100%, but this depended greatly on the criteria used. The largest series by Zhang et al. (10) reported control rates in acromegaly of 96% overall using a GH of less than 12 ng/mL as their definition of control. In studies using normalization of IGF-I as a criterion, control/cure was achieved in 20–70% of patients. Radiosurgery afforded excellent control of tumor growth—over 90% in most studies (9). Clearly, the rigorous use of modern criteria for hormonal control in acromegaly will be required in future studies to ascertain the true efficacy of radiosurgery.

ADVERSE EVENTS ASSOCIATED WITH RADIOTHERAPY IN ACROMEGALY

Adverse events in radiotherapy relate to radiation damage of normal structures. Older forms of radiotherapy that were relatively indiscriminate in the targeting of the delivered radiation dose were associated with brain necrosis. Milder forms of radiation-induced brain injury can manifest as deficits in cognition, memory, mood, and alertness.

Post-radiation damage can occasionally involve the visual pathways, and with external beam radiotherapy, it has been estimated to occur in about 2% of cases (1).

Hypopituitarism is a frequent finding in patients after radiotherapy. Adrenal, thyroid, and gonadal hypofunction have been reported to occur in 5–56%, 12–67%, and 11–67% of cases, respectively, during long-term follow-up of 5–10 years (1). In their recent 15 year follow-up study involving 47 acromegalic patients, Minniti et al. noted that hypopituitarism was common during long-term follow-up after conventional radiotherapy, increasing from 33% of patients at baseline to 57% at 5 years, 78% at 10 years and 85% 15 years after radiotherapy (4). Data on hypopituitarism after newer radiotherapeutic modalities for acromegaly are too scant to make a definitive determination of the risk of this adverse event during long-term follow-up. The rates of hypopituitarism following radiosurgery for patients with acromegaly are difficult to interpret as patients may have undergone surgery and previous radiotherapy.

Work from United Kingdom suggests that patients with pituitary adenomas (not limited to acromegaly) who are treated surgically and then receive radiotherapy have an increased risk of cerebrovascular mortality compared with the general population (11). In a cohort of 334 patients with pituitary adenomas treated between 1962 and 1986, 33 deaths due to cerebrovascular disease were noted, compared with 8 expected deaths. In contrast, Erfurth et al. reported no excess cerebrovascular mortality in a similar cohort of 342 patients with pituitary tumors treated between 1952 and 1996 (12).

Concerns about the risk of late-onset radiation-induced neoplasms have been raised. While reviews of data from external beam radiotherapy have identified only a handful of potential cases of second tumors among thousands of patients treated (13–15), the relative risk of developing a glioma and other tumor formation are greatly increased with the general population (15,16). Radiosurgery, on the other hand, has yet to be associated with definitive cases of radiation-induced second neoplasms, however, follow-up has been of a much shorter duration (9).

SUMMARY

Radiotherapy is a useful treatment option in selected cases of acromegaly where other therapies have failed. In patients with residual tumor that is not amenable to resection and cannot be controlled by medical therapy, radiotherapy may offer control of tumor growth. Hormonal control in acromegaly following radiotherapy is poor in the medium term and may take up to a decade to take effect. Given the increased mortality associated with poorly controlled acromegaly, medical therapy is warranted to control GH and IGF-I secretion in the interim period of years while waiting for radiotherapy to take effect. Hypopituitarism is common after external beam radiotherapy, although the corresponding data for radiosurgery are complicated by the fact that many patients have had previous surgery or external beam radiotherapy.

REFERENCES

1. Eastman RC, Gorden P, Glatstein E, Roth J. Radiation therapy of acromegaly. Endocrinol Metab Clin North Am 1992; 21(3):693–712.
2. Wass JA. Radiotherapy in acromegaly: a protagonists viewpoint. Clin Endocrinol (Oxf) 2003; 58(2):128–131.
3. Barkan AL. Radiotherapy in acromegaly: the argument against. Clin Endocrinol (Oxf) 2003; 58(2):132–135.
4. Minniti G, Jaffrain-Rea ML, Osti M, Esposito V, Santoro A, Solda F, Gargiulo P, Tamburrano G, Enrici RM. The long-term efficacy of conventional radiotherapy in patients with GH-secreting pituitary adenomas. Clin Endocrinol (Oxf) 2005; 62(2):210–216.
5. Brada M, Rajan B, Traish D, Ashley S, Holmes-Sellors PJ, Nussey S, Uttley D. The long-term efficacy of conservative surgery and radiotherapy in the control of pituitary adenomas. Clin Endocrinol (Oxf) 1993; 38(6):571–578.
6. Jalali R, Brada M, Perks JR, Warrington AP, Traish D, Burchell L, McNair H, Thomas DG, Robinson S, Johnston DG. Stereotactic conformal radiotherapy for pituitary adenomas: technique and preliminary experience. Clin Endocrinol (Oxf) 2000; 52(6):695–702.
7. Perks JR, Jalali R, Cosgrove VP, Adams EJ, Shepherd SF, Warrington AP, Brada M. Optimization of stereotactically-guided conformal treatment planning of sellar and parasellar tumors, based on normal brain dose volume histograms. Int J Radiat Oncol Biol Phys 1999; 45(2):507–513.
8. Milker-Zabel S, Zabel A, Huber P, Schlegel W, Wannenmacher M, Debus J. Stereotactic conformal radiotherapy in patients with growth hormone-secreting pituitary adenoma. Int J Radiat Oncol Biol Phys 2004; 59(4):1088–1096.
9. Laws ER, Sheehan JP, Sheehan JM, Jagnathan J, Jane JA Jr, Oskouian R. Stereotactic radiosurgery for pituitary adenomas: a review of the literature. J Neurooncol 2004; 69(1–3):257–272..

10. Zhang N, Pan L, Wang EM, Dai JZ, Wang BJ, Cai PW. Radiosurgery for growth hormone-producing pituitary adenomas. J Neurosurg 2000; 93(suppl 3):6–9.

11. Brada M, Ashley S, Ford D, Traish D, Burchell L, Rajan B. Cerebrovascular mortality in patients with pituitary adenoma. Clin Endocrinol (Oxf) 2002; 57(6):713–717.

12. Erfurth EM, Bulow B, Svahn-Tapper G, Norrving B, Odh K, Mikoczy Z, Bjork J, Hagmar L. Risk factors for cerebrovascular deaths in patients operated and irradiated for pituitary tumors. J Clin Endocrinol Metab 2002; 87(11):4892–4899.

13. Jones A. Radiation oncogenesis in relation to the treatment of pituitary tumours. Clin Endocrinol (Oxf) 1991; 35(5):379–397.

14. Bliss P, Kerr GR, Gregor A. Incidence of second brain tumours after pituitary irradiation in Edinburgh 1962–1990. Clin Oncol (R Coll Radiol) 1994; 6(6):361–363.

15. Brada M, Ford D, Ashley S, Bliss JM, Crowley S, Mason M, Rajan B, Traish D. Risk of second brain tumour after conservative surgery and radiotherapy for pituitary adenoma. Br Med J 1992; 304(6838):1343–1346.

16. Tsang RW, Laperriere NJ, Simpson WJ, Brierley J, Panzarella T, Smyth HS. Glioma arising after radiation therapy for pituitary adenoma. A report of four patients and estimation of risk. Cancer 1993; 72(7):2227–2233.

Index

About the Authors

Aart Jan van der Lely is the head of the Section of Endocrinology and the Clinical Research Unit of the Department of Internal Medicine at the Erasmus University Medical Centre in Rotterdam, The Netherlands. Dr. van der Lely's research interests include neuroendocrine disorders of the pituitary gland and the metabolic effects of neuroendocrine gut hormones.

Albert Beckers is Professor of Endocrinology at the Centre Hospitalier Universitaire de Liège, University of Liège, Belgium. Dr. Beckers' research focuses on the management of acromegaly and other pituitary diseases, MEN-I syndrome and endocrine cancer therapy.

Adrian F. Daly is a Research Fellow at the Department of Endocrinology, Centre Hospitalier Universitaire de Liège, University of Liège, Belgium, whose scientific research focuses on the epidemiology and outcomes of pituitary disorders.

Steven W. J. Lamberts is Professor of Medicine at Erasmus University Medical Center in Rotterdam, The Netherlands and is currently Rector Magnificus of Erasmus University. His long-standing research interests include the treatment of pituitary diseases, neuroendocrine tumors, glucocorticoid sensitivity and aging.

David R. Clemmons is Professor of Medicine and Chief of the Division of Endocrinology and Metabolism at the University of North Carolina at Chapel Hill, North Carolina, U.S.A. Dr. Clemmons' research interests include the physiological and pathological functions of insulin-like growth factors and their binding proteins and their clinical role in metabolism and nutrition.

Milton Keynes UK
Ingram Content Group UK Ltd.
UKHW050451071024
449327UK00015B/327